modern-day
macrobiotics

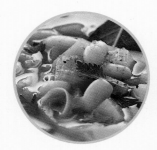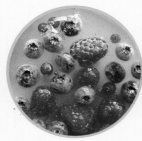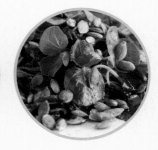

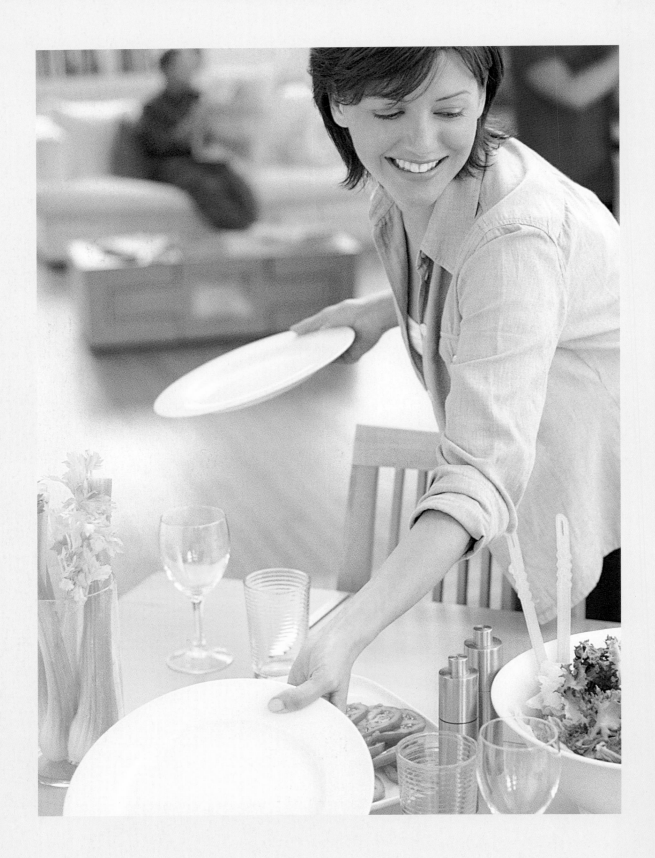

modern-day
macrobiotics

transform your diet and feed your mind, body, *and* spirit

SIMON G BROWN

North Atlantic Books
Berkeley, California

First published in 2005 in the United Kingdom by Carroll & Brown
Publishers Limited

This edition published in the U.S. and Canada 2006 by
North Atlantic Books
P.O. Box 12327
Berkeley, California 94712

Managing Art Editor Emily Cook
Cover designer Ayelet Maida
Photographers Jules Selmes, Will Heap, Winfried Heinze
Printed in Singapore

Modern-Day Macrobiotics is sponsored by the Society for the Study of Native
Arts and Sciences, a nonprofit educational corporation whose goals are to
develop an educational and crosscultural perspective linking various
scientific, social, and artistic fields; to nurture a holistic view of arts,
sciences, humanities, and healing; and to publish and distribute literature
on the relationship of mind, body, and nature.

Library of Congress Cataloging-in-Publication Data
Brown, Simon, 1957-
Modern-day macrobiotics : transform your diet and feed your mind, body,
and spirit / Simon G. Brown
p. cm.
Includes index.
ISBN-13: 978-1-55643-643-7 (pbk.)
ISBN-10: 1-55643-643-2 (pbk.)
1. Macrobiotic diet. I. Title.
RM235.B76 2006
613.2'64--dc22

2006024702

2 3 4 5 6 7 8 9 Star Standard 12 11 10 09 08

contents

the principles of **macrobiotics**

macrobiotics and health

the **macrobiotic** kitchen

macrobiotic menus

macrobiotic recipes for life

foreword by Michio Kushi

When I first met George Ohsawa in 1945, he was passionate about healing in the biggest sense of the word. He wanted to take the principles that worked so well for healing individuals and use them to heal a world that had been ravished by the Second World War. It was this idea of World Peace that inspired me to eventually join the macrobiotic movement.

At the end of the decade I went to America, joined later by my dear wife Aveline. By 1953 we were able to start simple classes, mainly for young people, in Boston, and six years later start the Erewhon the first natural food company in America.

During the 1960s my macrobiotic teaching attracted many free-minded, adventurous-spirited people who wanted to reach out to a different life, an alternative to the materialistic lifestyle that was leading people toward poor diets and, in some cases, poor health.

As time went by, my study houses evolved into a proper center and we managed to set up a network of macrobiotic centers throughout America and Europe where people could learn about the ideas behind macrobiotics and how to cook the foods. Whereas many of the original friends who came along were hippies, macrobiotics now started to appeal to all areas of society including doctors, healthcare professionals, actors, sportspeople, business people, and politicians. There was a huge growth in the movement and this was a time when I wrote many books and traveled the world carrying the dream of a better world through peace and health.

In the four decades that I have had the honor of dedicating myself to macrobiotics, my biggest joy has been in sharing in the success of each person who has found better health through the macrobiotic way of life, foods, and cooking. There have also been challenges, however, and my greatest sadness has been that we live in a world where there are still wars, killing, poverty, and preventable disease. There is still so much to be done.

I first met Simon in the 1980s when he assisted me with my consultations at macrobiotic summer camps. When he returned to run the macrobiotic center in London, he and his associates regularly invited Aveline and myself to give talks and we were able to continue our relationship working to promote macrobiotics, a message of health and peace.

I am very pleased he has used his experience to write this book and I wish all those who read it good health and the ability to lead a full and adventurous life.

Michio Kushi
Brookline, MA, USA

introduction

I was first introduced to macrobiotics in 1982 when my sister, Melanie, fell in love with a man who had been following a macrobiotic lifestyle for several years. Melanie went to macrobiotic courses at the Community Health Foundation in London and became a full-fledged enthusiast. We used to argue passionately about the philosophy behind macrobiotics, but I had to admit the foods seemed to be giving her more energy and her skin had a radiant, healthy appearance.

I had grown up with the feeling that my heart could be stronger, I had occasionally suffered palpitations and experienced pains in my chest. I had read enough to know that my current diet was far from ideal. Surprisingly for my age – I was in my early twenties – I experienced several acute attacks of gout around this time.

Melanie persuaded me to try a macrobiotic diet for three months. The deal was that if I did not feel better after that she would stop nagging me. I accepted her challenge and learned how to cook the foods.

Early days
At first the food was pleasant but a bit bland. I missed my sugary foods, breads, and desserts. However, as time went by, my enjoyment of these new foods increased and any longings for my old diet lessened. Within six weeks I noticed a gradual improvement in my health. I was surprised to find my digestion and bowel movements greatly improved, even though I was not aware of any problems before. My energy levels increased and where there used to be a heavy feeling, sometimes accompanied by a mild headache, I now felt lighter and freer. It was as though a great weight that was holding me back had been lifted.

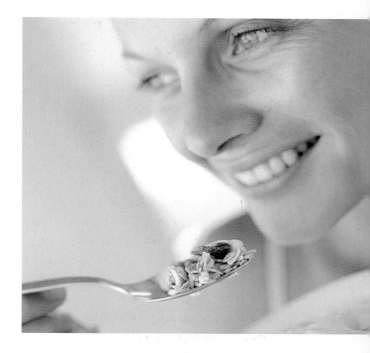

By the third month I had no recurrence of the gout and I felt more secure about my heart. Naturally, I continued and went to more classes, learning more about the ideas behind macrobiotic thinking.

Seeing the benefits
By this time Melanie had married Denny Waxman, a well-known macrobiotic teacher and counselor. In 1984 he asked me to join him in running a macrobiotic center in Philadelphia. I moved to America and immersed myself in a complete macrobiotic lifestyle, running courses, helping Denny with his counseling and, of course, continuing to eat macrobiotic foods myself.

There was a strong macrobiotic community in Philadelphia and I met many people who had recovered from all kinds of illnesses – arthritis, cancer, diabetes, asthma, eczema, migraines,

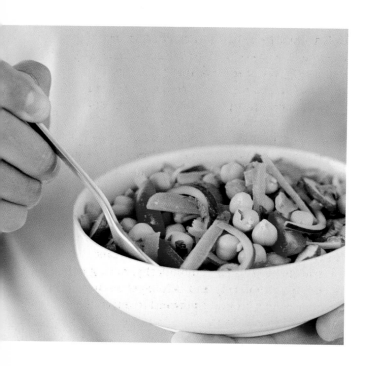

ovarian cysts, heart disease, digestive disorders. I was able to see firsthand the amazing healing powers the macrobiotic diet had. People who had been diagnosed with terminal cancer had managed to reverse the condition. Despite some cynicism about the concepts surrounding macrobiotics, I was still experiencing significant improvements in my own health while also witnessing the huge benefits enjoyed by others.

During this time, I was able to study with Michio Kushi, generally recognized as the world authority on macrobiotics. His lectures were always a revelation, I came out feeling my mind had been stretched and expanded in ways I did not think possible. I also used to assist him with his consultations, where I could see firsthand how he would design a specific macrobiotic diet for each person. I also enjoyed many cooking classes with Michio's wife,

a short history of macrobiotics

The word macrobiotics ("macro" meaning great and "bios" meaning life) was first used by the German doctor Christoph von Hufeland, who published his book *Macrobiotics: The Art of Prolonging Human Life* in 1796.

When his book was published in Japan, it is assumed that George Ohsawa, generally seen as the founder of macrobiotics, became familiar with von Hufeland's ideas while formulating his own philosophy on diet and health.

The search for balance
George Ohsawa had recovered from tuberculosis of the lung and colon in 1911, using a diet of whole, living, natural foods eaten in season, which had been recommended by Dr Sagen Ishizuka. Dr Ishizuka was a military doctor who, during the late-1800s, had had great success in helping many people recover from serious health problems. His theory was that the correct balance of potassium and sodium and acid and alkaline in the human diet leads to good health.

George Ohsawa was so grateful for his new lease of life that he dedicated the rest of his life to continuing Dr Ishizuka's work.

Spreading the word
The founding principle of macrobiotics is that each of us is responsible for our own life and health – and, at the time, this was radical and pioneering thinking. People lived their lives simply: when you were ill, you went to a doctor for medicine; there was little consideration given to diet and lifestyle. George Ohsawa traveled extensively, spreading his dietary message wherever he went. He ran courses and, in Japan, trained a group of students to go out into the world and spread the word of macrobiotics to other continents.

Five of his students, Michio and Aveline Kushi, Herman and Cornelia Aihara, and Shizuko Yamamoto, moved to North America; others went to France, Germany, and Brazil. Wherever they went, they popularized a huge range of Eastern ideologies,

Aveline, and twice a week helped cook macrobiotic meals for the 90 or so people that came to the center to eat.

In 1986 I was invited back to London to run the Community Health Foundation – Europe's largest natural health center at the time, with a macrobiotic clinic, teaching rooms, a cooking school, a food shop, a bookshop, and a restaurant. Here you could learn anything from t'ai chi to acupuncture. I was able to continue my connection with Denny Waxman, Shizuko Yamamoto and the Kushis as they became regular special teachers and counselors in London.

Macrobiotics for life
I started my own counseling practice and taught macrobiotic courses. It was around this time that I wrote a book with Dr Hugh Faulkner called *Against All Odds*, which charted Dr Faulkner's recovery from pancreatic cancer. He had been given three months to live, but through macrobiotics enjoyed another seven years of good health, eventually dying in his mid-80s.

Since 1993, I have continued to live a macrobiotic lifestyle, bringing up four boys and helping many others start their macrobiotic journeys. I was fortunate to be able to enjoy a successful career in feng shui, writing many books on the subject.

This book takes me back to my roots, and in it I wanted to share with you over 20 years' experience of eating macrobiotically, raising my family macrobiotically and helping thousands of other people around the world to enjoy the benefits of macrobiotics.

practices, and products in the West, pioneering the health food movement. Under their macrobiotic umbrella came shiatsu, Do In, nine-ki astrology, meditation, reiki, chanting, the *I Ching,* and oriental diagnosis.

East meets West
Macrobiotic centers and communities sprang up throughout America and Europe during the late 1970s, attracting people who wanted to learn about ki energy, yin and yang, the five elements, trigrams, and karma. There was a huge explosion of interest in everything from the East. Members of the macrobiotic community embraced acupuncture, aikido, and ta'i chi, helping them become established.

Inevitably, many macrobiotic ideas that were pioneering in the late 1970s and early 1980s were mainstream by the 1990s.

Food's healing power
However, more and more people started to turn to macrobiotics to help them recover from serious health problems. This turning point was largely fueled by a book called *Recalled by Life* by Dr Anthony Sattilaro, which charted his recovery from cancer.

Now the emphasis was on healing. As the success stories grew, the macrobiotic diet became know as a "cancer cure" diet. Its popularity with people recovering from cancer in turn meant that the diet became more purist, with the focus on clean, healing foods. This, however,

tended to put off people who were looking for a generally healthy lifestyle, and even gave the macrobiotic approach the reputation of being extreme, despite being broadly in line with recommendations from the World Health Organization.

Many of the foods associated with macrobiotics were hard to come by. However, now things have changed and many of the foods I'll be recommending are available in supermarkets.

My intention with this book is to show how macrobiotics can be incorporated into a healthy lifestyle, and how by changing your diet in small ways you can enjoy the benefits that good, healthy food – from a farm, not a factory – can impart to us all.

what is the macrobiotic diet?

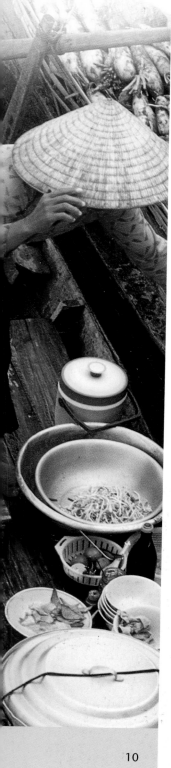

The ultimate healing diet, macrobiotics is a flexible, safe way of eating that helps you to find those foods that are right for you.

Food for health

The food we eat is one of the primary influences on our health, and because of this macrobiotics focuses on elements of the foods eaten by the world's healthiest societies. In fact, the macrobiotic diet excels in all measures of healthy eating: it is high in fiber; low in saturated fats; has a high mineral and vitamin content; and is high in complex carbohydrates. It uses ingredients that are low on the glycemic index, menus that are balanced in terms of sodium and potassium and acid and alkaline, and it incorporates a wide variety of ingredients and cooking styles.

Choose your style

Macrobiotics works on many different levels. You can use it to feed yourself more energy; to build a more healthy body; to improve your mind; or to experience greater emotional stability. You can also follow a macrobiotic diet for a short time to feel better; do it one day a week to keep your digestive system in good working order; try it for three months for more dramatic health improvements; or eat a macrobiotic diet for life.

Your choice over the foods you eat has an influence on you that goes far beyond whether you enjoy the taste. You really are what you eat, as all your cells are built on the food you eat, the water you drink, and the air you breathe. For this reason it is important to know how a food is likely to affect you in the long-term.

examples of healthy foods from around the world

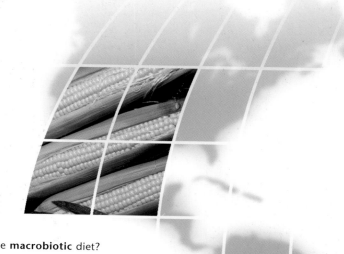

Macrobiotics clearly outlines how different ingredients, combinations, and cooking styles interact with your digestive system, influence your blood quality and, ultimately, build a healthy body and mind.

Body talk

One of the long-term goals of eating macrobiotically is to reach a point at which your body can begin to "tell" you which foods will be best for you.

Most of the time we shut out any connection between the food we eat and the more subtle influences it has on our bodies. However your body holds a "record" of all the various dishes you have eaten and of the way your body responded to them. It knows that every time you have something sugary, your blood sugar levels become elevated, leading to a period of heightened activity; and that every time you drink coffee, you become more acidic and lose fluids.

However by focusing more carefully on what you eat and how you feel, it is possible to bring that connection to the surface and use it to help you make the right food choices.

Whole, living foods

Very important in the macrobiotic diet, whole foods are still alive up until the point at which you cook them, and they retain a great deal of their living energy after cooking. This living energy interacts with your own energy and changes it as a result, making you feel different.

Whole foods also retain greater concentrations of nutrients, as opposed to processed factory foods, which oxidize, losing some of their goodness as a result.

When starting macrobiotics, it is helpful to experience a diet that is made up entirely of whole, living foods, such as brown rice, whole oats and barley, vegetables, beans, seeds, nuts, and fruit. And for general good health, I would recommend that at least half your foods should fall into this category.

AMERICA
polenta
corn on the cob

CHINA
noodles
green tea

INDIA
basmati rice
lentil soups
spices

JAPAN
miso
shoyu
tofu
sea vegetables

MIDDLE EAST
couscous
falafel

NORTHERN EUROPE
pickles
oats
natural breads
casseroles

SOUTHERN EUROPE
pasta
salads
hummus
olive oil
garlic
wine

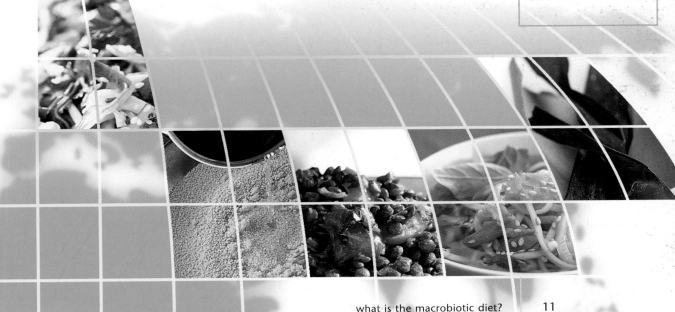

what makes macrobiotics special?

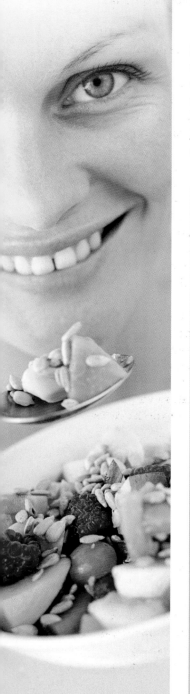

Because it has developed over almost a century, there have been plenty of opportunities to test macrobiotic theory and develop its full potential. It has evolved from a healthy, rural Japanese diet into one that can be applied anywhere in the world.

Safe and healthy

Over the years, macrobiotics has been placed under the microscope by each new theory on healthy eating and by all the new nutritional discoveries. But each time it has proved itself to be a safe and common sense approach

change your energy

There are many influences on your energy – the weather, other people, your home, the exercise you do – however food is one of the most powerful. Food has its own living energy and when you eat it you take this energy deep into your body, directly changing your own life-force from the inside. The food you eat not only changes your body on a biological level but also on an energetic one. Each meal has the potential to change the way you feel, your emotional state, and even your long-term attitude to life.

You can estimate the kind of life-force a dish has by looking at the way it grows, its growing season, where it grows, how it is processed, and the cooking method used. This means you can "design" a meal to change your own energy in a way that you think will be most helpful to you. For example, if you wanted to be more relaxed, you might choose something that grows in the autumn when the environmental energy is more settled, a food that has a round shape and that grows steadily. A sweet taste is also more relaxing, so you might choose a pumpkin or rutabaga, for example. If one of these was cooked slowly into a vegetable stew or soup you would have a dish that contains energy that spreads out evenly and slowly, helping your own energy flow in a relaxed manner. To feel more settled, you might add vegetables that grow down into the ground like carrots or parsnips.

This body of knowledge is unique to macrobiotics and is an important part of being able to create an individual diet that helps you feel the way you need to in order to get the most from your life.

12 reasons to choose macrobiotics

1   It is a broad, varied diet primarily consisting of grains, vegetables, fish, beans, seeds, fruit, and nuts.

2   Many people claim that eating a macrobiotic diet has helped them to recover from illness.

3   It is a flexible approach to eating that can be used over a few days or for life.

4   Using macrobiotic principles you can choose and prepare foods to change the way you feel.

5   You can eat anything as long as you know what the likely influence of that food is and are sure it will lead to good health.

6   The high fiber used in macrobiotics keeps your digestive system healthy.

7   Being low in saturated fats, a macrobiotic diet enhances your blood quality, improving your circulation and heart.

8   Low on the glycemic index, macrobiotic foods encourage even blood sugar levels, making it easier to lose weight and enjoy emotional stability.

9   The foods are well balanced in terms of acid and alkaline as well as sodium and potassium.

10   The predominance of complex carbohydrates means that the meals provide plenty of sustainable energy, leading to greater stamina.

11   The general macrobiotic diet is high in proteins, iron, calcium, and other minerals and vitamins.

12   Macrobiotics is a complete approach to healthy eating that encompasses everything from selecting good ingredients, to cooking methods and eating.

to healthy eating and healing. Its lasting – and growing – popularity prove that macrobiotics is no fad.

Living energy

George Ohsawa and later Michio Kushi developed the link between traditional Oriental medicine and macrobiotic foods. This builds on the idea that everything has a living energy. This is similar to the principles used in practices including acupuncture, t'ai chi, and yoga. This living energy – known as *chi* in China, *ki* in Japan, and *prana* in India – flows through our bodies, carrying our emotions, beliefs, and spirit. This energy or life-force influences the way we feel, our moods, and, ultimately, our health. So, in a similar way that you might use needles or herbs you can use the powerful healing life-force of food, which carries its energies and nutrients deep into your blood and onto every cell in your body (see box, left).

We all have to eat, so why not make each meal a healing experience for the body?

life-force food

Macrobiotics is a unique approach to healthy eating as it recognizes that every food has its own living energy and that this energy influences the life-force within us.

how to use this book

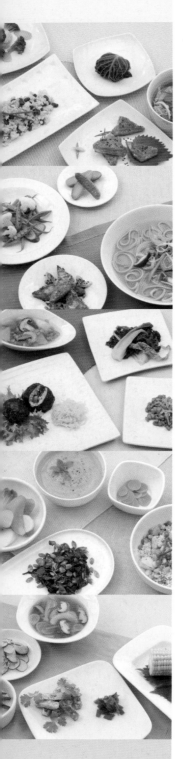

Whenever you start a new health regime, it is important to understand what you are doing and how it works. Of course, the biggest test is *whether* it works. If you increase your energy levels, lose excess weight, or recover from a health problem, that may be proof enough, but I would still recommend you research the process that took you to this happy conclusion, as knowledge and understanding put you in a more powerful position where you feel more in control of your own destiny. Part 1, The Principles of Macrobiotics, outlines how macrobiotics works and how it can help your body heal itself, why you can enjoy more stable emotions, how your energy levels increase, and why you will achieve a healthy weight.

The ingredients for health

When you start a new way of eating, it's common for those close to you to feel concerned – or sometimes even threatened. People still worry about not eating meat or drinking milk, even though evidence points to both being unnecessary and unhealthy in excess. In Part 2, Macrobiotics and Health, you'll find information on where various essential nutrients come from so you can feel confident within yourself and reassure others that what you are doing is safe.

One of the most daunting aspects of starting a new diet is getting to know new, perhaps different, foods. Part 3, The Macrobiotic Kitchen, takes you into the macrobiotic store cupboard and gives you information on where to find the various foods, how to store them, how to use them, and what they can do for you. This section also helps you to understand the qualities of the various foods so you can get a better idea of what you need most.

Design your diet

As macrobiotics is so flexible you can choose how to practice it. In Part 4, Macrobiotic Menus, I have included several menu plans, from a one-day detox to a four-month regeneration diet, all based on recipes to be found later in the book. It really depends on what you are looking for. Once you have decided on how you want to practice macrobiotics, you can use the recipes in Part 5 to get started.

To get you started, I suggest you use recommended macrobiotic dishes and menu plans in this book to eat a healthy well-balanced diet. However, the long-term aim of learning about macrobiotics is to have the knowledge and experience of eating macrobiotic foods to design your own diet: anything can be part of your macrobiotic diet as long as you know the effects of what you are eating. The goal is to be responsible for your own health and take the initiative to do whatever is necessary to enjoy optimum health.

Unless you are familiar with all the shortcuts, you could find yourself spending most of your day in the kitchen, which is not the aim at all. Macrobiotics is all about living a large life and therefore you need to balance the time spent on a way of eating to give you the levels of health you want and having the time to go out and enjoy your health. Eating a wide and varied diet of living, whole foods can be time consuming unless you plan ahead, and in Part 4, I have suggested various shortcuts for you to try. Part 4 also contains advice on how to prepare quick 10-minute meals and choose healthy foods when you eat out.

The right balance

To be successful with your food, you need to enjoy a wide variety of ingredients and cooking styles. This ensures you get the biggest range of nutrients and increase your ability to absorb them. The recipes in Part 5 will give you plenty of variety – but you must make an effort to try them all. It is human nature to learn a few favorites and use them again and again. I would highly recommend that you push yourself to try them all and keep going back to this part of the book to refresh your repertoire.

The recipes in each section are in the order of those you might use most to improve your health to those you might use more often to maintain your health or to make a transition into healthy eating. Each recipe has symbols to show you how a particular dish will move your energy (see box, right). In addition, there is a guide to how long a dish takes to prepare and cook along with the number of days it will keep if refrigerated. This is helpful as you can make enough of some dishes to last several days, greatly reducing the time you need to spend in the kitchen. I have also included notes on what each dish is good for.

MOVING YOUR ENERGY

Food is energy, and each type of food contains different energy that, as you eat it, can change your internal energy. In Part 5, each recipe has been assigned one of the following symbols, which equate to the energy that the food will impart. So, if you want to feel more relaxed, look for recipes with the flowing/relaxing symbol; if you want to feel a cleansing energy, look for the thinning/cleansing symbol, and so on.

 UP

 OUTWARD

 INWARD

 DOWN

 FLOWING/RELAXING

 THINNING/CLEANSING

Macrobiotics is all about balance, and to give you some indication of how balance is achieved, I've included photographs (see left, also shown on pages 16, 36, 54, 98, and 120) of five delicious macrobiotic meals, along with their percentage breakdowns. These are merely suggestions, but they do give some guidance on the mix of ingredients (and therefore nutrients) you should be aiming for for optimum good health.

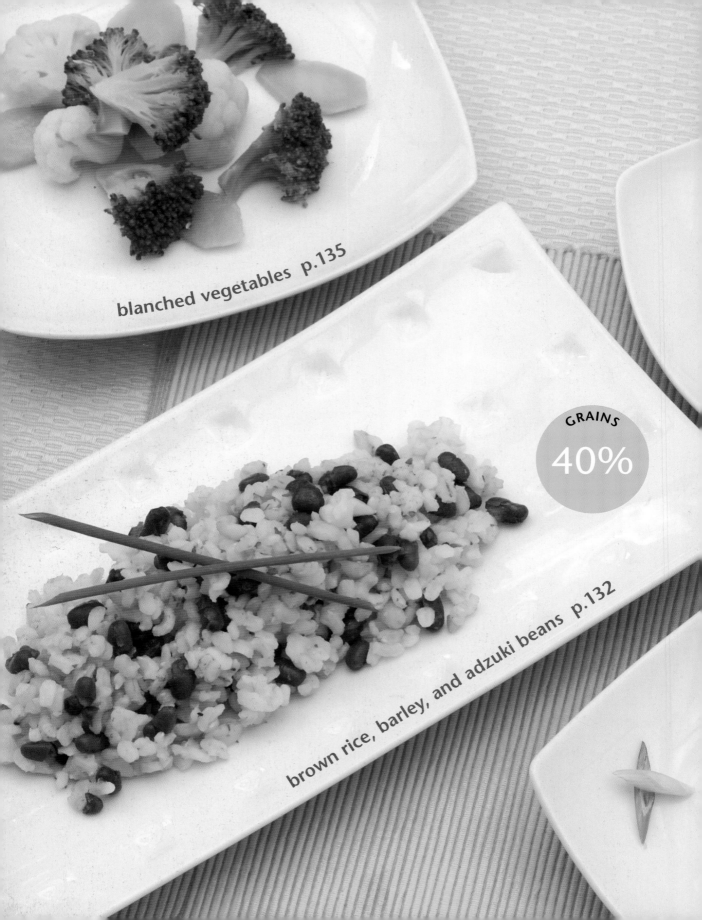

blanched vegetables p.135

GRAINS
40%

brown rice, barley, and adzuki beans p.132

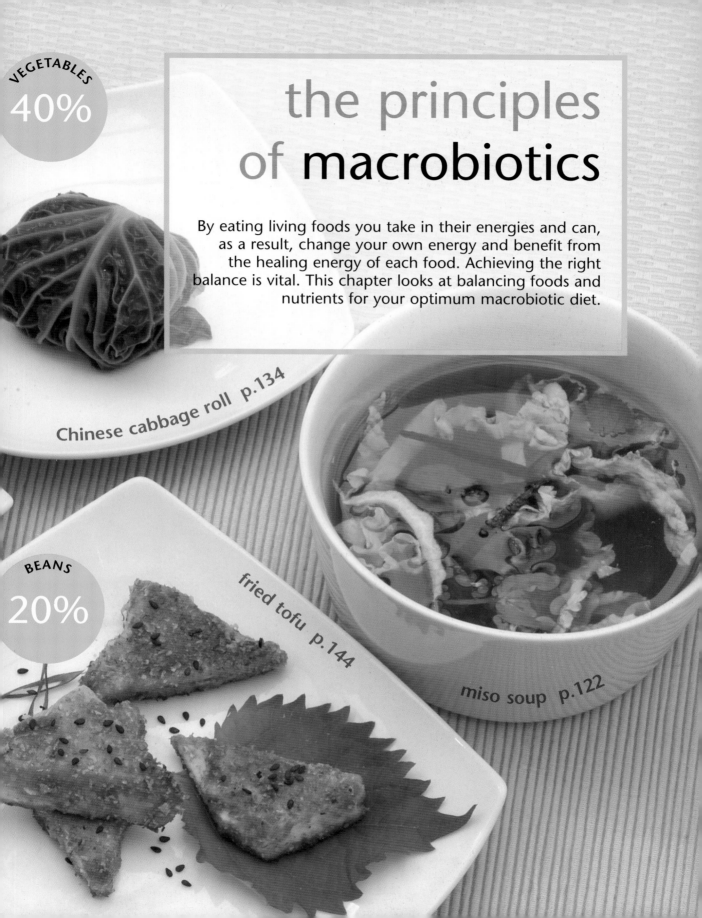

VEGETABLES
40%

the principles
of macrobiotics

By eating living foods you take in their energies and can, as a result, change your own energy and benefit from the healing energy of each food. Achieving the right balance is vital. This chapter looks at balancing foods and nutrients for your optimum macrobiotic diet.

Chinese cabbage roll p.134

BEANS
20%

fried tofu p.144

miso soup p.122

food is energy

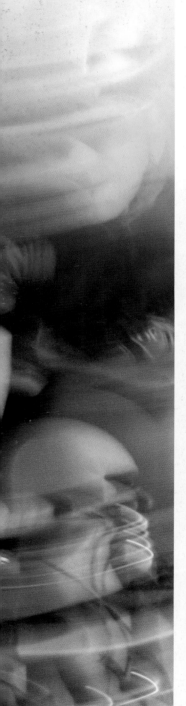

As you eat different foods you take in their energies, and these in turn interact with and change your own internal energy.

The resulting new energy may make you feel different emotionally; it may help you think differently; or it may help lift your spirits. The longer you eat foods with a similar energy, the deeper and longer-lasting this influence will be. Naturally, the energy from living foods is more beneficial than that from processed, adulterated foods.

What are living foods?
Living foods are those foods that can still grow. For example, if you put whole grains, dried beans, or seeds on a damp cloth in a dark cupboard they will sprout; fruits can be planted to grow into a new plant; root vegetables can be planted so that they grow again; leafy greens can be kept with

INFLUENCES ON THE ENERGY OF FOOD

The direction it grows	Up, down, spreading out, horizontal
The climate it grows in	Tropical, temperate
Its growing season	Spring, summer, autumn
Type of environment	Soil, air, or water
Its position in the growth cycle	Seed for new life or mature and fully grown
Where it grows	Mountains, flat lands, stony soil, trees, rivers, sea
Growth	Slow, fast
Its position within the evolutionary cycle	Primitive, modern
Local foods	Traditional, natural foods from your area

their stalks in water so that they continue to live; fermented foods have a micro process in which living enzymes flourish.

The energy of each food is the sum total of everything that has contributed to its growth. With living foods you can actually see this energy by using Kirilian photography.

Those foods that are no longer "alive" – such as fish, meat, and dairy products – still retain a living energy, but this will be less than that in foods that were alive up until they were cooked, and it will diminish with time. Likewise, processed foods will also have some energy, but this will be muted compared to living foods.

Changing your energy

It takes the body about 10 days to replace all its white blood cells, so eating foods with strong living energy for this period could have a significant influence on your well-being. In four months, the body changes all its red blood cells, so eating a healing diet for this period will lead to more profound changes. This should also be long enough to discover how your body feels at optimum health. Ultimately, you could rebuild your whole body based on a certain kind of energy, choosing your food according to the type of energy you want to promote.

The direction of energy in a meal

The directions in which different foods grow also influences the energy they impart. When you eat these foods, you will take in some of their directional energy, helping to move your own energy in the same direction. This is particularly true of vegetables. For example, greens such as leeks, scallions, or Chinese cabbage will help to move your energy up your body, making you feel slightly lighter, sending more energy into your chest and head. Root vegetables will encourage your energy to settle, helping you feel stronger in your lower abdomen. This helps take energy away from your head, making it easier to relax and be more down-to-earth and practical. Round vegetables help to gently spread energy out, giving you a warm, satisfying feeling around your stomach. Cooked grains help move energy inward, whilst foods that thin out your energy are cleansing.

Cooking styles

In addition to the ingredients, the style of cooking also influences the way your energy flows. Steaming will encourage energy to move up, sautéing encourages it to move outward, slow stewing to move down, pressure cooking to move inward, boiling to flow. You could, therefore, stew some carrots slowly to settle your energy, or steam greens to help your energy move up more actively.

When using food for healing, you can select ingredients and prepare them in a way that sends healthy, living energy into certain parts of your body. For example, you might steam spring greens to help overcome congestion in the lungs, or use fried onions to spread out energy, stimulating the periphery of your body. You can even use a combination of energies: to stimulate the mind, for example, I might suggest a miso soup with fried onions, Chinese cabbage and scallions. Some grated ginger would make the experience more intense.

Seasonal goodness

It was Sagen Ishizuka who first proposed that eating foods in season could have health benefits. He realized that in a temperate climate the different foods that become available in each season carry the energy and biological make up of that season and help you feel in harmony with the prevailing weather. This is most readily applied to fruits: strawberries ripen in the late spring; apricots and peaches become available in the summer; while apples and pears are ready in the autumn.

Certain vegetables – such as winter squash, parsnips, and asparagus – are still seasonal. Of the whole grains only corn-on-the-cob is obviously seasonal.

Over time, as you eat more and more foods when in season, you will begin to take in the energy of the seasons more strongly, making a more powerful connection with the rhythms of nature. This, in turn, encourages you to bend and adapt to the world in which we live, giving you greater harmony, and making you feel more flexible.

Climate considerations

It is also true that foods that grow naturally in certain climates are ideally suited to the people living in those climates. So, for example, eating predominantly tropical foods while living in a cold climate may not be ideal for your health: your blood might become too thin, or too acidic and lack fats. You may find that eating foods grown in the same climate in which you live enables you to feel more comfortable with the prevailing weather conditions.

Local foods

If you want to to strengthen the bond with your local environment, try eating more foods that grow locally. If the area in which you live has a long history of a healthy community enjoying longevity, you can assume that the traditional local foods will provide you with the ideal energy and sustenance to thrive. Conversely, if there is little evidence of long-term health benefits or, worse, a history of poor health in the region, it would be better to use some of the other influences on food listed on page 18.

THE DIRECTION VEGETABLES GROW

 UP

Leeks, scallions, Chinese cabbage, asparagus, collard greens, kale, broccoli, cauliflower, parsley, watercress

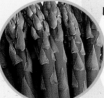

 SPREAD OUT

Onions, pumpkins and winter squash, rutabaga, turnips, cabbage, potatoes, sweet potato, radishes, ginger, garlic

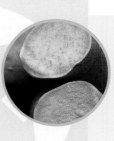

Air, soil, or water

The medium in which your food grows also has an effect on the energy you ingest. The parts of vegetables that grow above the ground – such as collard greens, broccoli, cauliflower, or scallions – will absorb more energy from the air, taking in a broader, changing energy, particularly if grown naturally, outside a greenhouse. They interact with the air and are stimulated by the sun; they experience changes in temperature; wind and rain; night and day.

Taking in more of this energy can help free up your spirits, making it easier to accept change and gain a broader perspective on the world.

Vegetables growing in the ground are nourished by a relatively stable environment. Carrots, parsnips, and radishes, for instance, are influenced by temperature and moisture, but these change comparatively slowly. To feel more settled and steady, try absorbing more of this energy.

Sea vegetables and fish take in the ebb and flow of the sea. They experience sunlight, night, and day but feel slow and small changes in

THE DIRECTION OF ENERGY IN COOKING

⬆	**UP**	Steaming
✖	**OUTWARD**	Sautéing
✳	**INWARD**	Pressure-cooking, pressing, baking
⬇	**DOWN**	Slow stewing
〰	**HORIZONTAL**	Boiling, blanching

temperature. In sea vegetables, this energy has an elastic quality, which will help you become more flexible, tenacious and adaptable.

Where and how the food grows

Where the food you eat grows will also play a part in the development of its individual energy. The carrot that has had to force its way through stony ground will have a different energy to one that has grown in soft, tilled soil. The former will have developed a tenacious and forceful energy, and if you eat this kind of

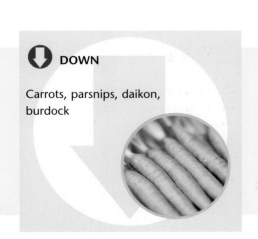

⬇ **DOWN**

Carrots, parsnips, daikon, burdock

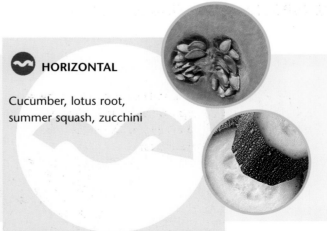

〰 **HORIZONTAL**

Cucumber, lotus root, summer squash, zucchini

carrot regularly, you will also pick up some of that energy. Try choosing twisted and asymmetrical root vegetables for greater strength.

Mountain vegetables, such as jinenjo, Japanese mountain yam, have a more hardy, vertical energy when compared to those growing on flat lands.

Fish, such as wild salmon, will have a very different energy to that of a squid. The salmon has to swim up stream, jumping waterfalls, while the squid floats in warmer waters. To fight your corner, you would benefit from taking in more of the salmon's energy whereas to relax you would be better with that of the squid.

Tree fruit, such as apples, plums, oranges, and lemons, grow high in the air. This exposes them to a very different energy to those that grow on the ground. Being further from the ground they carry an energy that could help you feel further removed from daily practical issues, enabling you to develop your imagination or to find a more lofty spirituality.

The growing cycle

Eating foods that are at the beginning of their growing cycle, such as beans, seeds, nuts, and whole grains, will

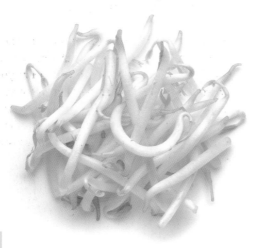

feed you with the energy associated with the beginning of life. This youthful energy is full of promise and that "anything can happen" spirit. It contains the energy necessary for growth and expansion. George Ohsawa placed great importance on retaining a sense of curiosity, the yearning to question everything like a child. He referred to it as "non credo" – literally meaning "believe nothing" or in other words, question everything. Eating grains and seeds will help you rediscover your sense of wonder and gain the enthusiasm to take on new challenges.

Foods such as vegetables, fish, and meat, particularly those that have not been farmed, factory processed, or grown in a greenhouse, are fully mature when eaten and bring with them an energy that has coped with survival. Taking in this energy, especially from wild fish or meat, increases the "fight-or-flight" mentality, sharpening your survival instincts. It also gives you the maturity to benefit from experience and a practical sense of wisdom.

With other foods, we only eat the part that feeds the seeds as they begin to grow. For example, the flesh of an apple is there to provide sustenance to the seeds: it is a kind of baby food. This, along with milk or milk products from cows or goats, gives us the kind of nourishment we needed during our first years of life. It is soothing, reassuring, and nurturing.

Growing times

The speed at which something grows will also influence its energy and, in turn, its effect on your energy. Radishes, squashes, zucchini, pumpkins, and cucumbers grow

EXAMPLES OF LIVING FOODS

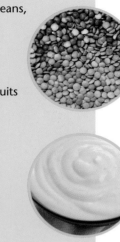

Whole grains	Whole oats, brown rice, wheat berries, millet, barley, corn-on-the-cob, whole rye
Dried beans	Lentils, adzuki beans, garbanzo beans, mung beans, kidney beans, pinto beans, navy beans, black or yellow soy beans, black-eye peas, lima beans, great northern beans
Vegetables	Leafy greens, root vegetables, sea vegetables
Fresh fruit	Berries, tree fruits such as apples and pears, ground fruits such as melons
Seeds	Sesame, sunflower, pumpkin, flax, linseed
Nuts	Almonds, filberts, walnuts, pecan, peanuts, cashew
Fermented foods	Miso, shoyu, vinegars, yogurt, soft cheeses, tempeh, natto, pickles

rapidly, tending to make quicker changes to your own energy. Slow-growing foods will have a slower but longer-lasting impact on your energy.

Primitive or modern?
Eating more primitive foods, such as sea vegetables, mussels, clams, or oysters, will feed your energy with more primitive stimuli. This is the energy of survival and reproduction, making these kinds of foods ideal for strengthening these instincts within you. Fermented food is another example of primitive food. The simple organisms in fermented foods will stimulate the most primal forces within you. These kinds of foods can be helpful when you simply want to enjoy the process of living.

Fruits are an example of more modern foods. Eating fruits can help elevate your thinking and enable you to take a greater interest in the future.

 foods to suit you

None of these ideas are to be taken as "all-or-nothing." The intention is not to eat local foods exclusively, nor does it mean you should only eat foods from your climate or when in season. You can try them exclusively for a while, to see how you feel, or simply use those principles that best suit your current needs. Once you have the benefit of experience, you can use macrobiotic principles as and when you need them.

acid and alkaline

The balance of acid- and alkaline-forming foods in the diet is key to good health, something that both Segan Ishizuka and George Ohsawa recognized very early on.

Acid versus alkaline

In a macrobiotic diet based on whole, living foods, the grains and some beans, such as lentils, are acid-forming, while vegetables and fruits are alkaline-forming (this is why it is important to eat as many vegetables as grains in a typical day). If you add in fish, dairy foods, and meat, your diet becomes more acid-forming, increasing the need for alkaline foods. Junk food, smoking, and alcohol make the diet even more acid-forming.

Sagen Ishizuka claimed that over-acidity generally led to poor health. When eating more alkaline-forming foods the body stores minerals. When your diet becomes too acidic, your body uses these stored minerals to redress the balance. Because minerals such as phosphorus are taken directly from the bones, this could lead to bone weakness and can aggravate arthritic conditions. A general acidic condition is also thought to increase the risk of cancer, headaches, and reduce your resistance to infection.

Achieving a good balance

It is much easier for the body to balance foods that are closer to neutral rather than trying to balance

MOST ALKALINE FORMING

Celery, dates, figs, herbal teas (most types), agar-agar, cantaloupe, watermelon, cayenne, lemons, limes, mangos, kudzu root, papaya, parsley, seaweeds, seedless grapes, watercress

MODERATELY ALKALINE FORMING

Beans (fresh, green), beetroot, broccoli, cabbage, alfalfa sprouts, bananas (ripe), almonds, apples, apricots, asparagus, collard greens, avocados, bancha tea, figs (fresh), carob, fruit juices, garlic, raisins, cauliflower, chard greens, daikon, dates, kiwi fruit, nectarines, passion fruit, peaches, ginger (fresh), grapefruit, kale, grapes, green tea, herbs (leafy green), lettuce (leafy green), pears, peas (fresh), peppers, pineapple, potatoes (with skin), pumpkin, radishes, raspberries, shiitake mushrooms, strawberries, squash, sweet potatoes, sweet corn (fresh), turnips, vinegar (apple cider) umeboshi plums, vegetable juices

SLIGHTLY ALKALINE FORMING

Olives, olive oil, artichokes (Jerusalem), eggplant, brown rice syrup, millet, miso, buckwheat, cherries, tangerines, chestnuts (dry, roasted), coconut (fresh), cucumbers, brussels sprouts, essene bread, goat's milk, honey (raw), leeks, mushrooms, okra, radishes, tomatoes, sea salt, onions, oranges, pickles (home-made), sesame seeds, shoyu, tofu, soy beans (dry), soy cheese, soy milk, spices, sprouted grains (most types), tamari, tempeh, vinegar (sweet brown rice) wild rice

the principles of **macrobiotics**

out extremes. And while it's not possible to create a balanced acid and alkaline diet from a list, it is possible to make sure your diet includes adequate sources of both.

Start by having roughly equal amounts of grains and vegetables and then try to match additional acidic and alkaline foods. For example, if you are eating more fish, reduce your intake of grains slightly and increase your intake of vegetables or fruits. Try having lemon or chopped almonds with your fish. If you enjoy coffee or alcohol, try also to eat more alkaline-forming foods.

To increase the alkaline-forming foods in your diet try a daily helping of miso soup with a variety of vegetables and sea vegetables; use more millet and reduce your use of other grains; have fresh melon for dessert; cook parsley as a vegetable dish; eat tofu instead of beans more often; drink kukicha (green twig tea) or herbal teas; have freshly squeezed vegetable or fruit juices.

The effects of everyday foods

It is difficult to produce a reliable table of acid- and alkaline-forming foods because some foods that appear acidic, such as lemons, actually result in a more alkaline condition in the body. Tomatoes, for example, are considered slightly alkaline-forming (and the riper the tomato, the more alkaline it becomes), but tomatoes become acid-forming where the stomach acid is low or the thyroid activity is abnormal – it depends on the health of your digestive system.

The table below gives you a broad guide to the acidity/alkalinity of many everyday foods, based on these foods' primary influence on the body.

NEUTRAL	SLIGHTLY ACID FORMING	MODERATELY ACID FORMING	MOST ACID FORMING
Cream, cow's milk, yogurt (plain), whey (raw) butter (unsalted), oils (except olive)	Eggs, kidney beans, pumpkin seeds, sesame seeds, barley, barley malt, butter, venison, spelt, spinach	Honey (pasteurized), blueberries, bran, cheeses, dry coconut, eggs, fish, fructose, oats, milk (homogenized), goat's milk (homogenized), rice milk, pasta (whole grain), grains (unrefined), dried beans (except soy beans), nuts (most except almonds), rye, ketchup, molasses (unsulfured and organic), maple syrup (unprocessed), mustard, pastry (whole grain), plums, popcorn (salted/buttered), potatoes (peeled), prunes, rice (basmati and brown), tea, wheat bread (sprouted organic)	White bread, pastries, and cakes (from white flour), chocolate, coffee, alcohol, carbonated soft drinks, fruit juices (sweetened), artificial sweeteners, beef, pork, poultry, fish, cereals (refined), cranberries, prunes, cream of wheat (unrefined), custard (with white sugar), yogurt (sweetened) flour (white wheat), ice cream, jams, lamb, maple syrup (processed), molasses (sulfured), pasta (white), peanuts, pickles (commercial), rice (white), seafood, sugar, table salt (refined/iodized), tea (black), walnuts, white vinegar (processed), whole-wheat foods

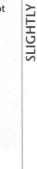

sodium and potassium

Sagen Ishizuka's research led him to conclude that the balance of the potassium and sodium salts in the body was the prime determinant of health, and that food is the main factor in maintaining this balance.

What are the benefits?
Eating a diet with a good balance of sodium and potassium will help your muscles and nerves to function properly (although those involved in intense physical exercise may require more potassium-rich foods). Your body will also be better able to maintain its ideal electrolyte and acid balance (see box, below).

Most people eating a Western diet consume far too much sodium, most of which comes from processed foods into which salts are added. One of the biggest risks of eating a high sodium diet is high blood pressure, which can lead to heart attacks, strokes, and kidney disease.

symptoms of potassium deficiency

- Muscle weakness
- Confusion
- Irritability
- Fatigue
- Heart problems
- Chronic diarrhea

Following a macrobiotic diet, you should find you have adequate sources of potassium while not taking in excessive sodium. Typical sources of sodium in the macrobiotic diet are salt, miso, shoyu (Japanese soy sauce), pickles, tekka (a mineral-rich powder made from root vegetables), umeboshi, and sea vegetables.

Good sources of potassium
Fruits and vegetables are good sources of potassium but, because potassium is water-soluble, these should be eaten raw or only lightly cooked (blanched for one minute or less, lightly steamed, or stir-fried). In the case of spinach, for example, potassium levels have been shown to drop by about 56 percent after blanching for several minutes. Alternatively, make a vegetable soup or a tea. Parsley tea, for example, will retain its potassium content in the liquid.

The salt balance
If your diet is too high in salt, you may experience cravings for more

electrolyte minerals

Potassium, sodium, and chloride comprise the electrolyte family of minerals. Called electrolytes because they conduct electricity when dissolved in water, these minerals work together closely in your body. Potassium is especially important in regulating the activity of our muscles and nerves. The frequency and degree to which our muscles contract, and the level to which our nerves become excitable, depend on the presence of potassium in the right quantity.

liquids, fruits, and desserts as your body tries to restore and maintain its proper balance. For this reason, if you are trying to lose weight or maintain stable blood sugar levels and avoid foods with a high sugar content, it is important to keep sodium-rich foods to a minimum.

However, it is also important not to have too little sodium in your diet, so regular, small amounts of sodium-rich foods should be eaten on a daily basis. This could take the form of a half teaspoon of miso in your soup; a pinch of salt with your cooked whole grains; a serving of pickles; a 2-inch strip of sea vegetable with your main meal; or a teaspoon of shoyu to season a dish. A few times a week, you could also sprinkle some tekka or shiso powder on your grains, or include olives and a pinch of umeboshi plum for seasoning. This is only a rough guide and you should reduce your salt intake if you feel tense, stressed, aggressive, have cravings for sweets, or suffer from high blood pressure.

Salt from the sea
When you do have salt make sure it is of good quality. Always try to use sea salt, and use a variety of sources as each kind of salt has different properties and imparts a different energy.

Because we evolved from the sea, taking in the energy of sodium-rich foods stimulates our deepest primal instincts. These foods stimulate our deepest biological memory and help us feel more in touch with the basic needs of survival and reproduction. Fermented sources of sodium-rich foods will bring in this energy more strongly, so use miso, shoyu, and pickles to increase this ancient energy.

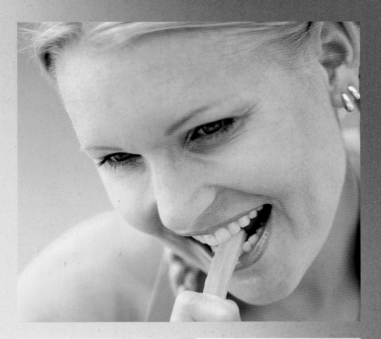

POTASSIUM-RICH FOODS

- Fruits and fruit juices
- Vegetables (fresh)
- Beef
- Whole wheat
- Brown rice
- Chicken
- Fish (fresh)
- Honey
- Yogurt
- Salmon (wild and fresh)
- Lamb
- Noodles
- Porridge oats/oatmeal
- Nuts
- Oysters
- Pasta
- Pork
- Scallops
- Seeds
- Shrimp
- Turkey

SODIUM-RICH FOODS

- Sea vegetables
- Salt
- Breads
- Butter
- Crab
- Ham
- Miso
- Cheese (except ricotta)
- Bacon
- Shoyu
- Tekka
- Clams
- Sauerkraut
- Corn chips or similar
- Umeboshi
- Ume-sprinkle
- Mustard
- Olives
- Pickled vegetables
- Sausage
- Tuna (canned)

glycemic index

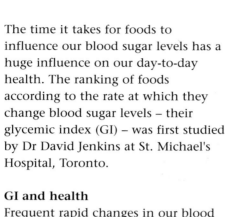

The time it takes for foods to influence our blood sugar levels has a huge influence on our day-to-day health. The ranking of foods according to the rate at which they change blood sugar levels – their glycemic index (GI) – was first studied by Dr David Jenkins at St. Michael's Hospital, Toronto.

GI and health

Frequent rapid changes in our blood sugar levels increase the risk of developing type 2 diabetes and can contribute to heart disease and strokes. Knowing which foods will maintain stable blood sugar levels is essential for anyone trying to control diabetes through diet. In addition, people often find that a rapid increase in blood sugar is followed by a rapid decrease, as the pancreas releases insulin so that the body reduces blood sugar levels by storing the excess sugars. This can result in cravings for more sugary foods, leading to dramatic blood sugar peaks and troughs throughout the day, a pattern that often leads to excess weight gain. People have found it is easier to lose weight by eating foods that encourage their blood sugar to rise slowly and gradually. However, it is possible to achieve a similar effect by simply eating a healthy diet of foods with a low to moderate GI.

The effects of high GI foods

There are, however, two other important issues, particularly from a macrobiotic perspective: the effect that the energy of these sugary foods has on our bodies, and the influence of unstable blood sugar levels on our emotions. As our blood sugar reaches a high, it is common to feel hyperactive, unfocused, and slightly out of control, while during a blood sugar low, feelings of depression and pessimism can take over. Rapidly changing blood sugar levels seem particularly to affect children, precipitating tears and tantrums, later followed by feelings of withdrawal.

glycemic index and glycemic load

The glycemic index (GI) is a system of measuring how different carbohydrate-rich foods act on blood sugar levels. The higher the number, the quicker the blood sugar response, so a low GI food will cause a slow rise, while a high GI food will trigger a dramatic spike, followed by a low. A GI of 55 or less is low, a GI of 56 to 69 is medium and a GI of 70 or more is high.

The glycemic load (GL) is another way to assess the impact of carbohydrate consumption that takes the glycemic index into account, but gives a fuller picture. A GI value tells you only how rapidly the carbohydrate component of a particular food turns into sugar. It doesn't tell you how much of the carbohydrate is in a serving of that food. You really need to know both to understand a food's effect on blood sugar. For example, the carbohydrate in watermelon has a high GI but as there is not a lot of it, watermelon's glycemic load is relatively low. A GL of 10 or less is low, a GL of 11 to 19 is medium and a GL of 20 or more is high.

6 interesting facts about the glycemic index

1 Whole grains have a lower GI than processed grains. For example, white rice has a GI of 64, brown rice 55.

2 You can greatly reduce the GI of brown rice by mixing it with whole barley.

3 Puffed grains, such as rice cakes or puffed rice cereals, have a much higher GI than the original whole grain.

4 The longer a food is cooked, the higher the GI. For example, spaghetti boiled in 0.7 percent salted water for 11 minutes has a GI of 59, whereas when it is cooked for 16.5 minutes it has a GI of 65.

5 Most vegetables have a GI that is too low to be considered significant.

6 Baking or sautéing foods raises their GI. Potatoes have a GI of 85 when baked, 75 when sautéd and 50 when boiled.

The ideal level

Maintaining stable blood sugar levels has long been an important aim of macrobiotic practitioners. Foods with a GI of 55 or less are considered ideal and looking through the chart on pages 30–31 you will see that most whole, living foods have a GI of 55 or less. The exceptions are millet, apricots, raisins, watermelon, broad beans, winter squash, beetroot, potato, sweet potato, and rutabaga.

However, another element to consider is the glycemic load (GL) of the food you eat, the amount of carbohydrate a food will convert into blood sugar. If the GL of a food is 10 or less it is considered low, so foods such as apricots, watermelon, broad beans, winter squash, beetroot, or rutabaga may increase your blood sugar quickly but do not raise it particularly far as there is not sufficient carbohydrate found in a typical serving.

 your body's response

The glycemic index is complicated and cannot be generalized to all people. Different people will have different reactions to food. Your body's response to food will vary according to several factors including: your age, activity level, insulin levels, the time of day, amount of fiber and fat in food, whether the food has been processed, what was eaten with the food, the ratio of carbohydrates to fat and protein, how the food was cooked, and your metabolism.

	Serving (grams)	GI (per serving)	GL (per serving)
Grains			
Baguette (white, plain)	30	95	15
Rye bread	30	50	6
White wheat	30	70	10
Whole-grain bread	30	71	9
Pita bread (white)	30	57	10
Muesli (Swiss)	30	56	9
Porridge whole oats	250	51	11
Porridge oat flakes/oatmeal	250	55	15
Barley, pot or pearled (whole)	150	25	11
Buckwheat	150	54	16
Polenta/cornmeal	150	69	9
Corn-on-the-cob	150	48	14
Millet	150	71	25
Rice (white)	150	64	23
Rice (basmati)	150	58	22
Rice (brown)	150	55	18
Rye (dry, whole)	50	34	13
Linguine (durum wheat)	180	46	21
Rice noodles	180	61	23
Spaghetti (white)	180	57	27
Spaghetti (whole-grain)	180	37	16
Rice cakes	25	78	17
Dairy			
Yogurt	200	36	3
Fruit			
Apple	120	38	6
Apricot	120	57	5
Banana	120	52	12
Grapes	120	49	9
Kiwi	120	53	6
Orange	120	42	5
Peach	120	42	5
Pears	120	38	4
Plum	120	39	5
Raisins	60	64	28
Strawberries	120	40	1
Watermelon	120	72	4

the principles of **macrobiotics**

	Serving (grams)	GI (per serving)	GL (per serving)
Juices			
Apple juice (unsweetened)	250	41	12
Carrot juice (fresh)	250	43	10
Orange juice	250	50	13
Beans (dried)			
Black-eye peas	150	42	13
Lima beans	150	31	6
Garbanzo beans	150	28	8
Haricot	150	38	12
Kidney beans	150	28	7
Lentils (brown, red, and green)	150	30	5
Mung beans/split peas	150	42	7
Pinto beans	150	39	10
Soy beans	150	18	1
Snacks			
Corn chips	50	63	17
Cashew nuts	50	22	3
Peanuts	50	14	1
Hummus	30	6	0
Sweetener			
Honey (pure)	25	58	12
Vegetables			
Broad beans	80	79	9
Peas	80	48	3
Pumpkin/winter squash	80	75	3
Sweet corn	80	54	9
Beetroot	80	64	5
Carrots	80	47	3
Potatoes (baked)	150	85	26
Potatoes (boiled)	150	50	14
French fries	150	75	22
Sweet potato	150	61	17
Rutabaga	150	72	7

This chart uses glucose as its reference. Glucose = 100. Many vegetables – artichokes, asparagus, avocado, broccoli, cabbage, carrots, cauliflower, celery, cucumber, eggplant, green beans, peas, leeks, lettuce, mushrooms, olives, onions, peppers, spinach, squash, tomato, yam, and zucchini, for example – have a GI of less than 55.

nutrition

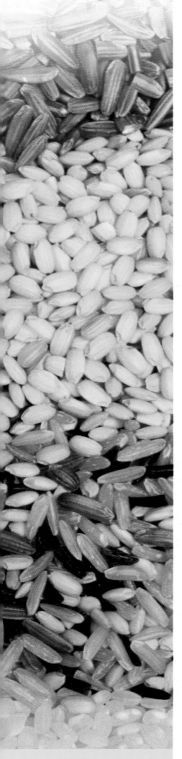

Many people mistakenly believe that the macrobiotic diet cannot provide them with the essential nutrients they need for long-lasting good health. And, while it's true that to have a healthy diet you must have a variety of foods in the right proportions, there is no reason why this can't be achieved with macrobiotics. The following tables show the amounts of each nutrient found in different foods and compare them to the US Food and Drug Administration's daily value (DV) reference points, devised to help consumers understand a food's nutritional content.

Protein
People starting out on a macrobiotic diet are often concerned about where their protein will come from. This is largely because it is assumed that all protein comes from meat. The fact is that all natural foods contain protein, otherwise they would not grow. Vegetables, grains, and beans are all high in protein (see box, right). As a macrobiotic diet is predominantly made up of these whole, living foods, supplemented with fish, it can actually contain more protein than other diets based on junk food, sugar, and processed foods. There has been some debate over whether protein from meat is of a higher quality, however leading medical opinion no longer supports this view.

Protein is comprised of 23 amino acids, of which we require just 10 to maintain proper health and vitality. Fish, eggs, meat, and dairy foods contain all 10 essential amino acids, while individual plant foods do not. Therefore, to get all the essential amino acids from a vegan-style macrobiotic diet it is important to have a daily mix of foods high in protein. Most typically this would consist of a mix of grains and beans or bean products. For example, a bean soup and a meal with brown rice in the same day will provide a complete range of essential amino acids. Seeds, nuts, and vegetables will also help ensure you take in all the essential amino acids on a daily basis.

Protein requirements are at their highest when exercising vigorously, for a child during a growth spurt or during pregnancy.

The World Health Organization recommends a minimum of 32 g of protein per day for a 68-kg (150-lb) man. The US Food and Drug Administration (FDA) recommends a higher level of 50 g per day.

Iron
Iron is an essential component of hemoglobin, the substance in red blood cells that combines with and carries oxygen around the body, and plays a vital role in many metabolic reactions. Iron deficiency is the most common mineral nutritional deficiency. It can lead to anemia, which is caused by low levels of hemoglobin in the blood, which in turn results in fatigue, dizziness, and low mood. External signs are a pale color on the inner lower eyelids, pale lips, or pale fingernails.

the principles of **macrobiotics**

As with protein, it is often assumed that meat is the best source of iron, however many green, leafy vegetables have three times more iron per calorie than that found in red meat (see box, page 34). For example, a sirloin steak has 1.9 mg of iron per 100 calories, whereas turnip greens have 6 mg of iron per 100 calories. The FDA daily value for iron is 18 mg.

At times of high demand, such as during pregnancy or blood loss from excessive menstrual flow, it may be necessary to increase your iron intake. A handful of parsley, steamed or sautéed in olive oil with dulse seaweed and a handful of pumpkin seeds eaten daily will help.

Calcium

It is normally assumed that the best source of calcium is dairy foods. Although dairy foods are high in this mineral, many other foods contain similar amounts. Unfortunately, dairy foods are also very high in saturated fats – the very thing that we are being urged to cut down on to improve our health.

Calcium in a macrobiotic diet primarily comes from vegetables, sea vegetables, fish, tofu, nuts, seeds, and small quantities of dairy foods. The recommended DV for calcium for adults between 19 and 50 is 1,000 mg.

Vitamin B_{12}

This vitamin helps to maintain healthy nerve cells and red blood cells. A vegan-style macrobiotic diet could be lacking in vitamin B_{12}, which can lead to pernicious anemia. Although vitamin B_{12} can be found in fermented products such as beer, miso, or tempeh, the quantities are too small to make a difference, so if

PROTEIN

	g/100 g	% of DV 50 g
Grains		
Barley	12	24
Corn-on-the-cob (boiled)	7	13
Millet	11	22
Oats	17	33
Rice, brown (medium)	8	15
Rye	15	29
Wheat (hard red spring)	15	30
Vegetables		
Broccoli tops	3	5
Kale	3	6
Leeks	2	3
Shiitake mushrooms (dried)	10	19
Parsley	3	5
Peas	5	10
Watercress	2	4
Beans		
Adzuki	20	39
Kidney	24	47
Garbanzo beans	19	38
Lentils	28	56
Natto	18	35
Peas, split	25	49
Soy	36	72
Tempeh	19	37
Tofu (hard/nigari)	13	25
Fish		
Shrimp	20	40
Cod	18	35
Haddock	19	37
Mackerel	20	40
Monkfish	14	28
Salmon (wild)	20	39
Tuna (bluefin)	23	46
Clams	13	25
Mussels	12	23
Seeds		
Pumpkin	25	49
Tahini	17	34
Sesame	18	35
Sunflower	23	45
Nuts		
Almonds	21	42
Hazelnuts	15	29
Peanuts	26	51

IRON

	mg/100 g	% of DV 18 mg
Grains		
Barley	3.6	20
Corn-on-the-cob	2.7	15
Millet	3.0	16
Oats	4.7	26
Rice, brown (medium)	1.8	10
Rye	2.7	14
Wheat	3.6	20
Vegetables		
Broccoli	0.7	4
Chard (Swiss)	1.8	10
Kale	1.7	9
Kelp sea vegetable	2.9	15
Leek	2.1	11
Parsley	6.2	34
Peas	1.5	8
Wakame sea vegetable	2.2	12
Beans		
Adzuki	5.0	27
Kidney	6.7	37
Garbanzo	6.2	34
Lentil	9.0	50
Natto	8.6	47
Soy	16	87
Seeds		
Pumpkin	15.0	83
Sesame	14.6	80
Sunflower	6.8	37
Tahini	9.0	49
Nuts		
Almonds	4.3	24
Hazelnuts	4.7	26
Fruit		
Raisins (dried)	2.6	14
Fish		
Clam	14	77
Grouper	0.9	4
Mussels	4.0	21
Oyster	6.7	37
Tuna	1.0	5
Squid	5.3	29
Meat		
Beef steak (porterhouse)	2.0	10
Chicken	1.1	6

you are concerned about your B_{12} intake, you should eat fish and seafood – the best sources of the vitamin – regularly. The body stores a few years' supply of B_{12} in the liver so it is possible to eat a vegan-style diet for several months before needing to build up your reserves again. Pregnant women and breastfeeding mothers have increased demands for B_{12} and young children may not yet have built up a store of B_{12}.

The daily value (DV) for vitamin B_{12} is calculated at 6.0 micrograms (ug). A food providing 5 percent or less of the DV is a low source; 10–19 percent of DV is a good source; and 20 percent or more is a high source.

Vitamin D

Vitamin D is absorbed through sunlight or certain foods. Although in many countries sufficient vitamin D may be obtained solely from sunlight, in countries where there are long periods of cloud cover, dietary sources are important.

Typical dietary sources of vitamin D are dairy foods, eggs, liver, and fish. In a macrobiotic diet, fish (see box above, right) and sunlight are the primary sources. The greater your exposure to sunlight, the less fish you will require. The daily value (DV) for vitamin D for adults is 400 IU.

VITAMIN D

	ug/100 g	% DV 400 IU
Sardines	500	140
Salmon	360	90
Mackerel	345	90
Tuna	200	50

VITAMIN B$_{12}$

	ug/100 g	% DV 6 ug
Clam	49.4	824
Egg	1.3	21
Herring	10.0	166
Mackerel	8.7	145
Salmon	3.2	53
Tuna	3.8	62
Mussels	12	200
Octopus	20	333
Oysters	16	266
Shrimp	1.2	19
Lamb	2.5	41
Pork bacon	0.7	11
Pork ham (cured)	0.9	14

CALCIUM

	mg/100 g	% of DV 1000 mg
Grains		
Oats	054	5
Vegetables		
Chinese cabbage	105	10
Kale	135	13
Kelp	168	16
Mustard greens	103	10
Parsley	138	13
Turnip greens (boiled)	190	19
Watercress (raw)	120	12
Wakame	150	15
Beans		
Kidney	143	14
Garbanzo (boiled)	105	10
Mung	132	13
Natto	217	21
Soy	277	27
Tempeh	111	11
Tofu hard (nigari)	345	34
Seeds		
Sesame	975	97
Tahini	426	42
Sunflower	116	11
Nuts		
Almonds	248	24
Hazelnuts	114	11
Dairy food		
Cheese, Brie	184	18
Cheese, Camembert	388	38
Cheese, feta	493	49
Egg	053	5
Milk, fresh whole	113	11
Yogurt, plain whole milk	121	12

Fiber

A macrobiotic diet is a great source of fiber. A high-fiber diet encourages regular healthy bowel movements and increases the speed at which food moves through your colon, which will ensure your digestive system is kept healthy and reduce the risk of associated cancers. You can test the time taken by swallowing fresh corn kernels whole and seeing when they appear in your stools. Ideally, they will appear within 48 hours. Someone on a low-fiber diet can find it takes up to two weeks for the corn to appear.

Fats

A macrobiotic diet is low in the saturated fats that may make your blood sticky and may eventually lead to heart and circulation problems. Most of the fats in the macrobiotic cupboard are mono-unsaturated, which have beneficial effects on cholesterol, while the remaining polyunsaturated fats provide useful nutrients.

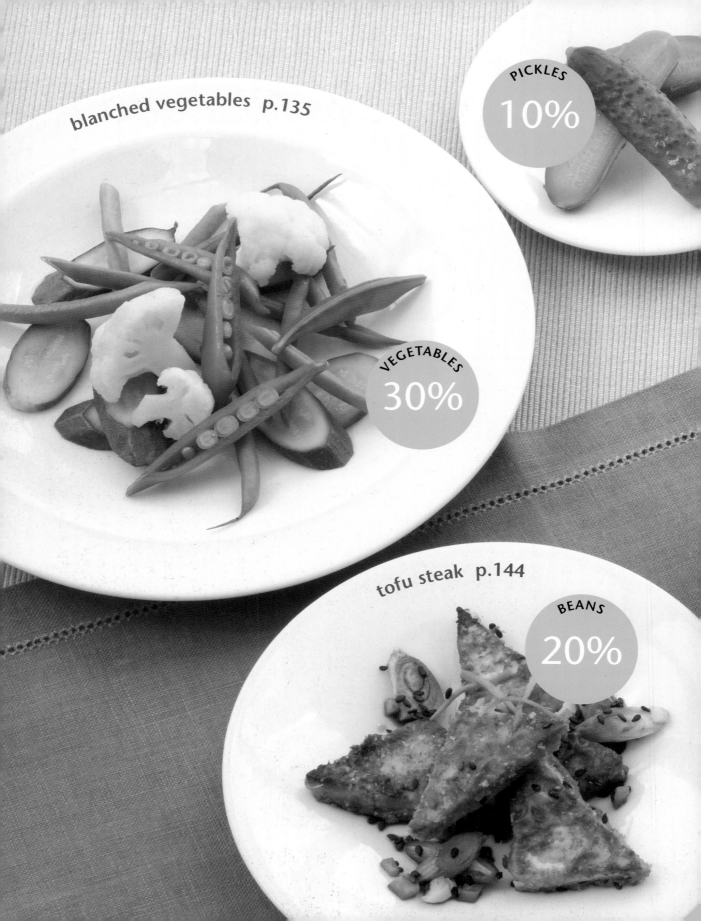

blanched vegetables p.135

PICKLES
10%

VEGETABLES
30%

tofu steak p.144

BEANS
20%

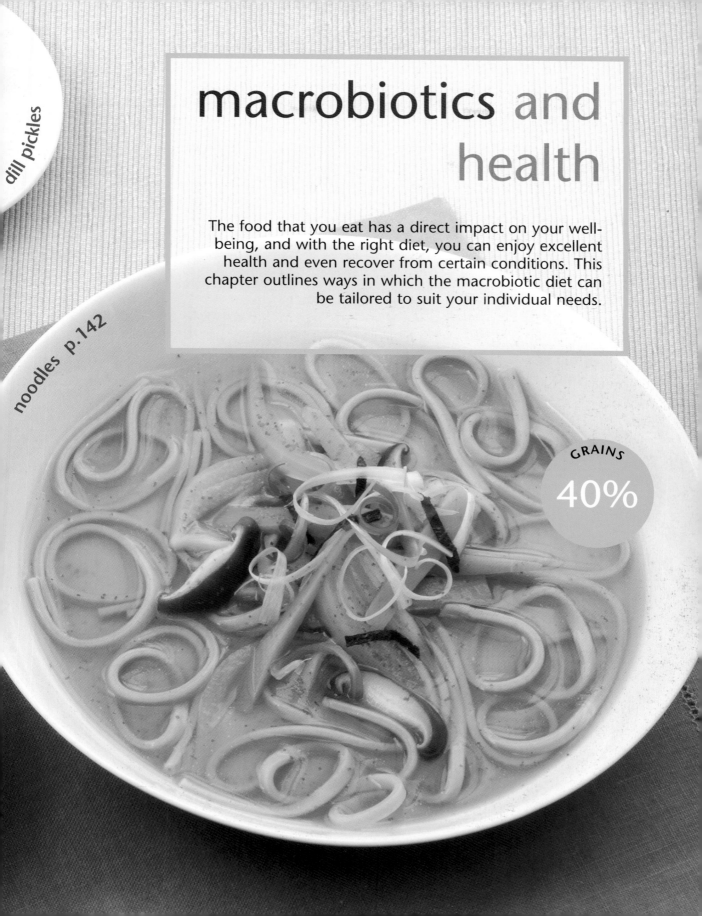

dill pickles

noodles p.142

macrobiotics and health

The food that you eat has a direct impact on your well-being, and with the right diet, you can enjoy excellent health and even recover from certain conditions. This chapter outlines ways in which the macrobiotic diet can be tailored to suit your individual needs.

GRAINS

40%

macrobiotics for general good health

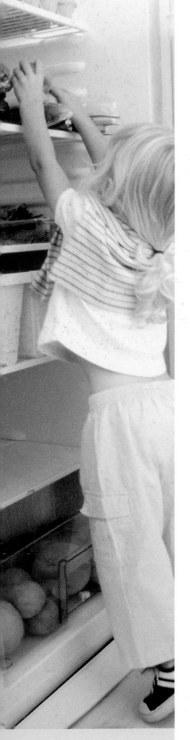

If you enjoy good all-round health, you can help to ensure that you continue to do so by adopting macrobiotic ideas. One of George Ohsawa's definitions of good health was to have the freedom to eat anything, bearing in mind the long-term effect of eating each food.

This doesn't mean that you should simply reach for anything marked "healthy" in the supermarket. Some of the modern "health" foods, such as soy milks and margarines, for example, have not been around long enough to demonstrate any health benefits and might even contribute to health problems in the long-term.

The easiest way to ensure you achieve a healthy, balanced diet is to eat foods that have a long and proven history of being eaten by the world's most healthy societies.

Your food, your way

Macrobiotics is not a "prescriptive" diet. Your own version of a macrobiotic approach will be unique to you. The best way I can illustrate this is by describing what I do myself.

I try to ensure that most of my foods are whole, living foods. In order to benefit from the different energies foods can bring, I eat a mixture of foods that grow in different directions – roots, green, and round vegetables – and use a variety of different cooking styles each day. Most of my foods come from a temperate climate, but I do have some tropical fruits and juices. Whenever I can, I like to eat fruits and vegetables in season and, in a typical day, I try to have a mixture of foods that grow in the air, in soil, and in water. If I have the choice, I would rather eat roots that have had to force their way through wild soil.

the concentrating process of toxins

Whenever we eat "second-hand" food we risk consuming higher levels of toxins. For example, if a cow eats food that has been treated with pesticides, the toxins that the cow cannot get rid of will be stored inside its body. Over time, if the cow continues to eat these foods, these stored toxins will become more and more concentrated. If you then eat the meat of this animal, you will also take in some of these toxins and, as the cow found them hard to eliminate, you are likely to find it hard to get rid of them, too.

Recent studies found that farmed fish can also contain a cocktail of toxins, including dioxins, PCBs, and pesticides, many of these building up as a result of environmental pollution – industrial chemicals and pesticides the use of which may be banned but which persist in the environment.

For me, it is easier to focus on what you need to eat for good health rather than worry about what not to eat. My own maxim, and one I have used to bring up my children, is that as long as we eat the essentials for good health each day – what I call the "core healthy foods" – then anything else is fine. It is only when other foods upset the balance to the extent that I no longer want to eat these core healthy foods that I need to get back to a more simple macrobiotic diet.

I have adopted all the macrobiotic principles and used them to develop a broad-based diet that is varied and interesting without being fanatical.

Core healthy foods

These vary between individuals, and I can only tell you what I put on my shopping list and would generally recommend to others. My list would include regular miso soups, whole grains, fresh vegetables, beans, seeds and herbal teas (see pages 118–119 for a more detailed plan.)

Along with these basic ingredients, I would include fish, fruits, dairy foods, nuts, juices, alcohol, and desserts. This second group of foods come and go depending on how I feel and my circumstances. I may, for example, eat fish every day for a week and then not at all for a month.

Are there things I shouldn't eat?

It is important to decide if there are any foods you do not want to include in your macrobiotic store cupboard. For example, I do not eat meat, although I know some people who eat a macrobiotic diet and feel better eating a little meat from time to time. If you are going to include meat in your diet, my advice is to make sure it

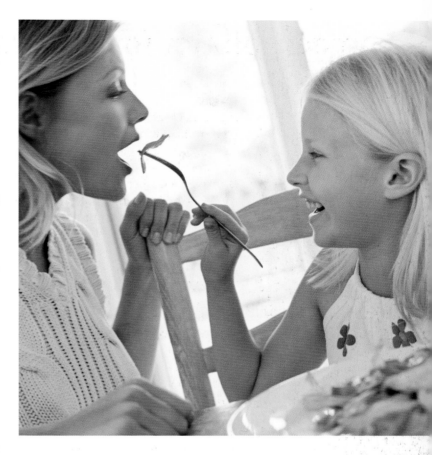

is organic. Similarly, I would not eat farmed fish and I would be cautious about non-organic dairy foods.

I also avoid irradiated foods, genetically modified foods, and those with additives and preservatives. I am also concerned about the explosion of new processed soy-based foods such as soy milks, ice creams, creams, and yogurts. I find these hard to digest – and the overuse of soy could lead to new intolerances. For similar reasons, I would not eat margarines as I am not convinced that the mix of oils most commonly used in their manufacture is healthy.

In all the above cases these are new foods, or conventional foods processed in new ways and the long-term effects of eating them are not yet

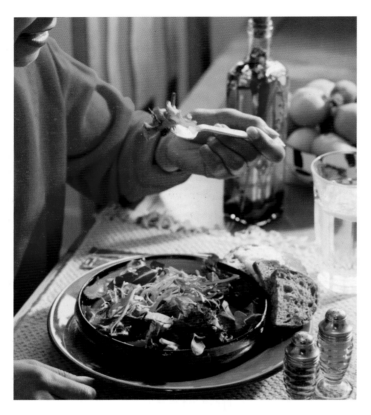

known. However, none of these new processes is solely motivated by creating better health: the prime motivation is increased profits.

Variety is everything

Traveling makes it possible to experience the different energy of local foods all over the world. In France and Italy I like a healthy Mediterranean diet of pasta, salads, and seafood; in Switzerland rosti and apple strudel; in Cape Verde tuna fish is a must. Similarly, when eating out, I like sushi, noodle dishes, and tiramisu. I use these examples to show that macrobiotics is not an "all or nothing" diet and it is perfectly possible to lead an ordinary, social lifestyle and travel while still eating your core healthy foods.

Inevitably, when eating out the range of foods I enjoy is much broader and this contrasts with a more stable routine at home. It is all about balance. Home is where it is easier to connect with organic, whole living foods and tune into the rhythms of nature.

Intuitive eating

Your body has an amazing capacity to guide you to the foods you need most on a physical and emotional level. You have stored information on all the meals you have eaten in the past and can subconsciously correlate this with the way you felt after eating that particular food.

One of the aims of eating macrobiotically is to reach a point where your body can intuitively tell you what to eat. Over time, you will gain the sensitivity to know from one mouthful of food whether it is good for you and whether it engenders the feelings you crave.

Physical cravings

All of us experience cravings from time to time, "messages" from our bodies telling us to address nutritional imbalances. Too many sodium-rich foods, for example, can result in a craving for more potassium-rich foods. Sugary foods that precipitate the overproduction of insulin and a consequent sugar low, will result in a craving for more carbohydrates to bring the blood sugar levels back up.

It's important to act on these cravings, and you should work out what the food you crave offers you. If it is not something you want to eat, look for a more healthy alternative. For example, you could substitute tahini for butter; you could try chewing your grains more to further break down the carbohydrates for sugar; you could try sautéed tofu instead of cheese. Each of these will satisfy your craving on a nutritional level.

You are less likely to get physical cravings if you are eating a wide variety of foods prepared using a range of cooking styles. Most physical cravings come from eating a diet that is too narrow and restrictive.

Emotional cravings

Emotional cravings occur when certain foods trigger deep-rooted emotional associations. For example, if as a child you were given ice cream as a reward or treat, you might find you can relive those happy emotions simple by eating ice cream. This becomes self-perpetuating, as every time after you eat ice cream, you will relive those feelings, thus increasing the strength of the association. You can use these emotional associations to make all your experiences with food more pleasurable. Whenever you eat healthy foods, surround yourself in a happy atmosphere. Put on your favorite music, watch a DVD that makes you laugh, eat with people who make you feel good, place fresh flowers on the table, do whatever it takes to really feel good while enjoying your macrobiotic foods.

the profit motive

In an effort to maximize yield and profitability, some farmers around the world use high-intensity farming methods – with minimum space for animals to grow and roam freely, factory farming methods, and the use of growth-accelerating hormones. The basic idea is to get your product, whether chicken, salmon, or cattle, to market as quickly as possible with the least cost. Because these conditions are so unhealthy there is a high risk of the spread of infection, making it necessary to feed the animal or fish on antibiotics to keep them alive until they are ready for slaughter. Needless to say, they are fed the cheapest food available that will encourage the quickest growth. Mad cow disease – with its disastrous consequences – came about because farmers were feeding cattle with the remains of other cattle. Recent European legislation bans the use of hormones and other chemicals, but evidence suggests that some unscrupulous producers still rely on these methods to maximize profits.

We all have to ask ourselves this: "is this something I want to take into my body?" It is not only the risk from the toxins involved, but also, do I want the energy of an animal that has lived in a cage and then gone through the process of mass slaughter to become part of me? There is no roaming the wild to develop a survival instinct for these animals, just anxiety, stress, and fear.

a macrobiotic healing diet

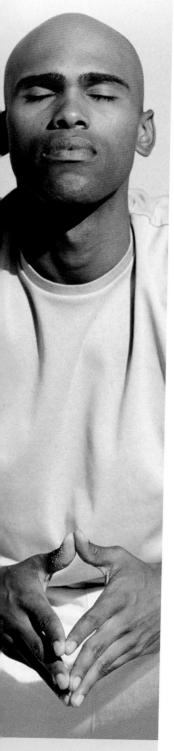

Macrobiotics has focused on food and health for over 200 years, enjoying varying degrees of popularity throughout this time.

Macrobiotics in action

In recent years, Doctor Anthony Sattilaro's book *Recalled by Life*, which recounted his own fight against cancer and the extraordinary recovery he underwent after embarking on a macrobiotic diet, precipitated a huge interest in using macrobiotics as a remedy for all kinds of illnesses.

Around the same time, other cancer sufferers were also experiencing amazing results that defied their medical prognosis. One man with whom I worked closely was Dr Hugh Faulkner. At the age of 74, Dr Faulkner was told that he had three to six months to live after being diagnosed with pancreatic cancer. He started to eat a macrobiotic diet and lived a full and highly active life for another seven years, as documented in our book *Against All Odds*.

I was in Philadelphia working with Denny Waxman, one of Dr Sattilaro's macrobiotic counselors, when Dr Sattilaro's amazing story hit the newspapers. Later, I was running a macrobiotic center in London when Doctor Faulkner's story was the subject of a great deal of publicity. Both times I was able to work directly with those seeking help, and eventually I became a macrobiotic counselor myself.

The following healing diet is based on my years of experience of working with thousands of people and seeing what works and what does not.

How does the healing diet work?

We already know that the human body has amazing powers of recovery. We can subject ourselves to terrible diets of junk food, live in polluted environments but still live a normal life for many years. People have recovered from serious illnesses as a result of all kinds of intervention – from a change of belief system or faith, to positive thinking, the help of a healer, conventional medicine, or macrobiotics. In all these situations, some kind of interaction takes place that resulted in the individual's powers of recovery turning unhealthy cells into healthy ones.

From a macrobiotic perspective, if a poor diet contributes to poor health, the obvious remedy is to replace the foods most likely to cause poor health with those most likely to result in good health. Eating foods with the optimum levels of nutrition and taking in healthy energy with your foods will lead to a healthy digestive system, good-quality blood, and an active immune system that will create the best environment to support the body's recuperative powers.

The macrobiotic healing diet can be combined with other forms of hands-on healing, faith-based healing, spiritual practices, positive thinking, and conventional medicine. It complements any other form of health care. However, although macrobiotics mixes well with diets based on food combining and those that use the glycemic index, it can be confusing if you try to mix different philosophies.

With macrobiotics, the theory is that the best diet to bring about healing is one that is low in fats, high in vitamins and minerals, based on complex carbohydrates, and which does not have excessive proteins. At the same time, it is important to achieve a good balance of acid and alkaline (see pages 24–5) and sodium and potassium (see pages 26–7).

First steps to health

To find out the extent to which macrobiotics can help you overcome a health problem, you will have to embrace it wholeheartedly and eat nothing but macrobiotic healing foods for four months.

It can be difficult to commit to this all at once. If you prefer to take things more slowly, you could start by using macrobiotic principles in their broadest form, incorporating new foods little by little.

If you are determined to make the change, the first task is to clear out all your cupboards, refrigerator, and freezer, and replace your old foods with the healing foods listed on pages 46–8. Again, you don't have to do this all at once, you can set your own timetable for the gradual transition to a complete macrobiotic diet.

There are other things to think about as you move toward a macrobiotic healing diet. Can you arrange your social life around eating at home? Could you reorganize your morning routine so that you can prepare and carry macrobiotic foods with you to work or when you go out in the evening?

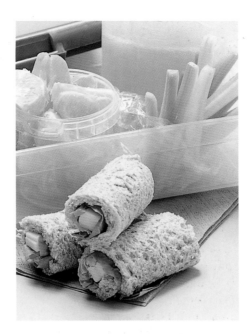

Many people who have been successful in recovering from health problems have researched macrobiotics and thought through the logistics of changing their diet to the point where they know they can make it work – and then go for it 100 percent.

Taste

Depending on what types of foods you are used to, when you start your healing diet some of the foods can taste bland. Like all our senses, our tastebuds need time to adjust, so it may take a few weeks before your tastebuds become sensitive to your new foods. You may need to be patient and accept that it may take some time before you really start enjoying your healthy foods.

Some foods, like miso or natto, can be an "acquired" taste so it is helpful to persist in including them in your diet – in small quantities – until you get used to them. Always remember, no one food is essential, so if you do

4 components of a macrobiotic healing diet

1 Low in fats – Too many fats make your blood sticky. If this results in platelets sticking together, you will not take in as much oxygen with each breath. In addition, if these fats are not burned off, they are stored in your body and can become sites for toxin storage, leading to poor blood circulation and the development of unhealthy cells.

2 High in vitamins and minerals – Essential for good health, the best ways to achieve a good vitamin and mineral intake is by eating a wide variety of fresh, organic vegetables and fruits.

3 Based on complex carbohydrates – Complex carbohydrates, particularly from whole foods, tend to break down slowly, leading to more even blood sugar levels. This reduces both the strain on the pancreas and the risk of sugar-related illnesses such as diabetes.

4 Ideal levels of protein – High protein levels have been associated with kidney problems. Also, as protein is key to the rapid multiplication of cells, high protein intake has been linked with the promotion of unhealthy growths in the body.

not manage to acquire the taste, don't worry, leave it out of your diet and try something else.

Simple and varied
The secret to using macrobiotics for healing is to get the basic diet right. There is no point worrying about special macrobiotic teas or which energy direction you need to emphasize if you have not got the foundations in place.

A healing diet is essentially made up of all the whole, living foods, but it is the variety of the foods you eat that will make the diet work and keep you interested. In a typical month, it is essential that you eat all the different whole grains, 30 or so different vegetables, at least six different beans, all the recommended seeds, a variety of fermented foods and various seasonings.

Just as important is the variety of cooking styles used. Each time you cook something, the way you cook it will influence and energy of the food and make certain nutrients more available (see box opposite for a list of the cooking styles and the way they influence the direction of energy.)

How long should I stay on a healing diet?
This style of macrobiotic eating is generally suitable for four months to a year at the most, but after that you will need to bring in other foods, particularly fish and processed grains. Once you have achieved a good level of health, start to broaden out your diet to include more macrobiotic foods (see pages 38 and 118.)

The recipes starting on page 120 are arranged so that the ones most appropriate for healing are listed first.

Check your mineral balance
Throughout your healing diet, take time to review pages 24–5 to ensure that you are eating sufficient alkaline-forming foods, and pages 26–7 for foods that are rich in potassium. It is possible for the healing diet to become too acidic and sodium-rich, both of which are believed to aggravate health problems.

Often, a mineral imbalance will result in food cravings (see pages 104–5), so adjusting your intake of certain foods can help redress this.

Feelings of tiredness, depression or low mood, lethargy or dreaminess can be due to a diet that is lacking in healthy sources of sodium or minerals. On the other hand, too much sodium often results in tight stiff muscles, headaches, constipation, and dryness.

Over-acidity is often cited as the cause of inflammation of the stomach, stomach ulcers, and aggravating all stress-related health problems, as the body secretes more acids when under stress. It is even thought that over-acidity can contribute to the formation of unhealthy cells and increase the risk of cancer. However too few acid-forming foods in the diet risks more fats being deposited in the blood, which can lead to your blood becoming too thick.

With this healing diet, you will consume a minimal amount of saturated fats and avoid an excess of sodium-rich foods, so reducing the need for the acid-forming foods and their potentially harmful effects. Maintaining this balance is key to healing.

Using the direction of energy
You can focus the beneficial effect of certain food into specific parts of your body by choosing particular vegetables and cooking styles (see also pages 19–21). The wholesome living energy of the vegetable will interact with your own life-force, improving the quality of your energy. In cases of serious illness this will make it easier for your body to turn unhealthy cells into healthy ones. Putting this concept into practice is very simple.
Lung Problems If you have a problem with your lungs, eat vegetables that grow upward – such as leeks, scallions, asparagus etc. – and steam them, enouraging the energy of the dish to move up your body. You can combine different types of energy to create a specific influence on your own energy. For example, if your lungs are congested, you might also want to move energy out by adding some thin slices of lotus root to your meal. To make the influence of the dish more powerful, add some grated ginger. Parsley tea is also helpful in breaking down congestion. If you look at parsley, it grows up and then out sharply, the ideal energy for breaking up mucus.

COOKING STYLES AND THEIR EFFECTS

Here is what happens to a carrot using different methods of cooking.

Boiling You will lose some of the water-soluble vitamins but retain the oil-soluble vitamins.

Steaming Similar to boiling except the loss of water-soluble vitamins is slower.

Sautéing Some of the oil-soluble vitamins will be lost but not the water-soluble vitamins.

Baking Increases the absorbable fat content of the carrot and raises the GI.

Stewing The carrot becomes sweeter and the carbohydrates are more accessible.

Pressure-cooking Increases the water temperature before boiling, exposing the carrot to a higher temperature, losing more of the fragile vitamins but increasing the availability of carbohydrates.

HEALING FOODS

These are typical foods you might use in the healing diet. The lists are ordered with foods you might use most often at the top and those that you will use less often toward the bottom of each section.

Whole grains
These should make up about 40 percent of your daily food by volume
- Brown rice – short-grain for cold weather, medium- or long-grain for hot weather
- Barley
- Whole oats
- Corn-on-the-cob
- Wild rice
- Wheat berries
- Whole rye
- Sweet brown rice

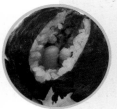
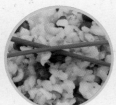
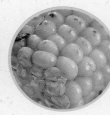

Vegetables
These should make up about 40–50 percent of your daily food intake. Ideally, eat a mixture of vegetables incorporating upward, outward, downward, and horizontal energies. The following list is for a temperate climate. In particularly hot weather, add more tropical vegetables.

 UPWARD ENERGY
- Broccoli
- Collard greens
- Chinese cabbage
- Kale
- Leeks
- Watercress
- Cauliflower
- Bok choy
- Celery
- Scallions
- Green beans
- Snow peas
- Peas
- Parsley
- Chard
- Asparagus
- Shiitake mushrooms

 OUTWARD ENERGY
- Onion
- Cabbage
- Radishes
- Ginger
- Garlic
- Pumpkin/winter squash
- Rutabaga
- Turnip

 DOWNWARD ENERGY
- Carrot
- Parsnip
- Mooli/daikon
- Burdock
- Kuzu
- Jinenjo

 HORIZONTAL ENERGY
- Cucumber
- Lotus root

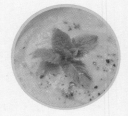
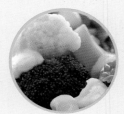
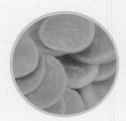
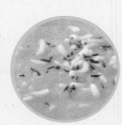
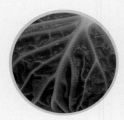

Sea vegetables
- Wakame
- Kombu
- Nori
- Dulse
- Arame
- Hiziki
- Agar-agar

Beans
These should make up about 10–20 percent of your weekly volume.
- Adzuki
- Lentils – green or brown
- Black soy
- Kidney
- Yellow soy
- Black-eye
- Pinto
- Navy

Seeds
Have one or two tablespoons most days.
- Pumkin
- Sesame
- Sunflower

Fermented foods
Use several of these every day.
- Miso – one teaspoon daily
- Shoyu – three to four teaspoons daily
- Umeboshi vinegar – three to four teaspoons most days
- Brown rice vinegar – three to four teaspoons most days
- Sauerkraut – one heaped tablespoon every other day
- Dill pickles – one or two most days

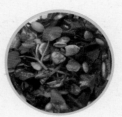

- Homemade pickles – one tablespoon most days
- Natto – one packet once or twice a week
- Takuan – pickled daikon – six thin slices once or twice a week
- Umeboshi plums – one per week

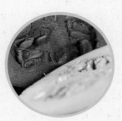

Seasonings
Use in small quantities to season foods.
- Sea salt – use in cooking
- Ginger – to season soups and stews
- Garlic – with fried foods or to season soups and stews
- Lemon – squeeze over fried foods or vegetable dishes
- Shiso powder – sprinkle a quarter teaspoon over grains occasionally
- Tekka – sprinkle a quarter teaspoon over grains occasionally
- Gomasio – sprinkle a teaspoon over grains occasionally

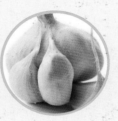

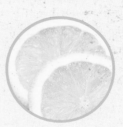

Oils
Use in cooking in cold weather and raw in hot weather.
- Olive
- Sesame
- Sunflower (raw only)
- Flax/linseed (raw only)

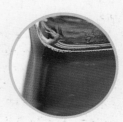

Fruits

Reduce to a portion of fruit once or twice a week – cooked in cold weather – and increase during hot weather.

- Apples
- Pears
- Raisins
- Plums
- Berries
- Olives (use as a part of a meal)
- Melons
- Grapes
- Apricots
- Peaches
- Cherries
- Tangerines/clementines
- Cherry tomatoes (use as a vegetable occasionally – once or twice a month)

Processed Foods

Use occasionally for convenience if necessary.

- Couscous
- Mochi
- Tofu
- Tahini
- Hummus
- Tempeh

Sweeteners

Ideally, do not use these at all as they will upset your blood sugar balance, however, if you crave greater sweetness, these are better than sugar or artificial sweeteners.

- Brown rice syrup
- Barley malt
- Natural corn syrup
- Maple syrup
- Honey

Teas

Drink a tea daily.

- Bancha/kukicha
- Green and roasted rice
- Peppermint
- Camomile
- Green
- Hot water and lemon

Juices

Best in hot weather. Can heat up the fruit juices or mix with boiling water to make them more relaxing.

- Vegetable juices
- Apple
- Pear

Alcohol

Not normally recommended for healing, although one or two glasses of red wine per week can be useful as an antioxidant and in reducing fats in the blood. Better in drier weather.

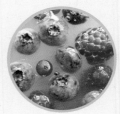
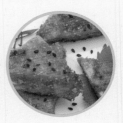
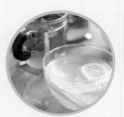
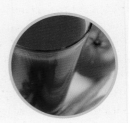
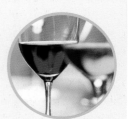

Cold symptoms For a cold you might want to try something with plenty of minerals, such as a miso soup, but to ensure that the energy moves up to your head, cook the miso soup with "up energy" vegetables, such as leafy greens, and then add some scallions toward the end of the cooking time. Similarly, you could make a bancha tea and pour it over chopped scallion and a teaspoon of shoyu to lift the beneficial effect of the alkaline tea and gain the fermented survival energy of the shoyu.

To relax your middle organs, stomach, liver, and pancreas, use round vegetables. You can encourage the relaxing energy by slowly cooking them until soft. When you eat this dish, you should feel a gentle, satisfying, relaxing feeling emanating from your stomach. This is helpful if you are someone who suffers from nervous tension. You could absorb a similar energy by boiling round vegetables such as cabbage, pumpkin/winter squash, rutabaga, and onions, or whichever combination is available, for 10 to 20 minutes, and drinking the juice.

If you want to drive the energy into your body, increasing your inner strength, try eating pressure-cooked grains, such as brown rice and barley, or cooking stews in a substantial pot with a heavy lid. To bring the energy out to the periphery of your body, add garlic, ginger, and oil. Frying the rice will be even more effective.

For greater strength in your intestines, bladder, bowel, or legs, use more downward-growing vegetables in casseroles. Again, to drive the healing energy deeper, cook slowly in a solid, heavy pot and combine with pressure-cooked grains at the meal. If,

for example, your intestines are tight or you are constipated, you will want to combine the downward energy with more outward and flowing energy. Here, it would be better to quickly boil carrots for more horizontal energy along with a vegetable like cabbage, which has more outward energy. For a bladder complaint, use a mineral-rich miso soup but include root vegetables so the healing energy moves down your body to your bladder.

In general, heated foods, drinks, and soups will project their energy into your body more strongly. The heat excites the energy of the food, helping it spread out and making it more active. In addition, the warmth will help relax you from the inside, making you more accepting of new energies. Liquids have the fastest effect on your body's energy, so use teas and light soups for quick results.

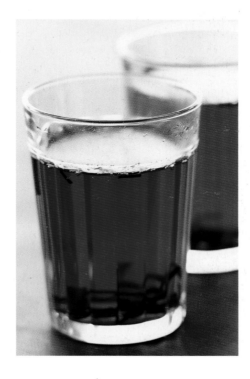

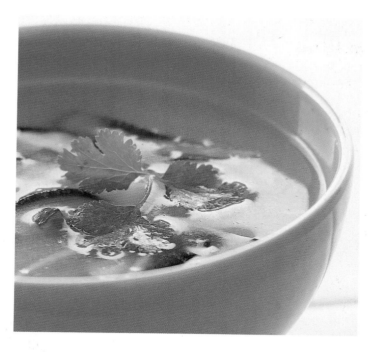

Using these simple principles, you can design your own remedies for any situation and try them out for yourself. With experience, anyone can take greater control over his or her own healing process.

From the roots to the tops

When eating a whole, living foods diet, try to include as much of the food as possible. As long as you buy organic foods there should be no need to remove the skins of vegetables or fruits. In the case of root vegetables, include the very tip of the root in your cooking. You can also include the top of the root, where the greens begin. Each part of the vegetable has useful nutrients and, eaten as a whole, will bring a more complete energy into your body. Try blanching radishes with their green tops, putting scallions – with their roots – in a soup, or boiling carrots with their tops for 10 minutes to gain the energy of the vegetable in its totality.

When to eat

It is also important to eat at regular times. After a while, your body will settle into a rhythm, knowing when to expect food and when to relax. Eventually, you will begin to secrete digestive juices in preparation for each meal as you get close to the appropriate time. The advantage of this is that you will find it easier not to eat between meals.

As with all the natural world, our bodies are made up of rhythms – night and day, seasons, lunar cycles, breathing, heartbeat, menstruation and so on. Any kind of rhythm creates a momentum that makes it easier to do more with less effort. Think of dancing to the rhythm of the music. By eating at regular times, you will set up another rhythm, making it easier to eat well and make the most of your food.

When you eat foods, even those with a moderate GI (see pages 28–31) there is a risk you will precipitate instability in your blood sugar levels, making it much harder to eat well for the rest of the day. This is a common complaint in people trying to lose weight. In this situation, try making your first meal of the day as late as possible. Even then, make sure that it is something with a very low glycemic index rating, such as a miso soup.

Likewise, if later you need to eat something sweet, leave it until as late in the day as possible – have a dessert after your evening meal, for example – so that by the morning your blood sugar will have regained its stability. Personally, I feel fine missing breakfast and eating two meals a day with a snack in the afternoon. Everyone is different and you will

USING FOODS FOR SPECIFIC HEALING

The following are examples of how you might use the living energy of foods to help specific problems.

To relieve a headache at the front of your head
• Miso soup with wakame and leafy greens – rich in minerals with "up" energy from the greens.
• Bancha tea with umeboshi and scallions – the tea and plums reduce acidity and the scallions move energy up.

To relieve a headache at the back of your head and ease a stiff neck
• Hot apple juice – the heat is relaxing and the energy of the apple is up and out.
• Steamed greens with sauerkraut – the sauerkraut helps reduce stickiness and thin your blood, while the greens move energy up.

For a cold
• Bancha tea with shoyu and scallions – the tea is slightly alkaline, the shoyu adds minerals and enzymes and the scallions move energy up.
• Hot ginger and lemon tea – the lemon rises and cuts through the mucus, while the ginger moves energy out.
• Miso soup with leafy greens – the greens move the healing energy of the soup up.

For a sore throat
• Fresh ginger, celery, and carrot juice – the ginger moves energy out, the celery moves energy up, and the carrot takes energy down, away from the throat.
• Hot lemon and rice syrup or honey – the lemon creates a local condition in the throat that subdues the growth of bacteria, while the syrup soothes the throat.

For congestion in the lungs
• Steamed greens and ginger – the steamed greens move energy up and the ginger moves energy out.
• Parsley tea – the parsley moves energy up and out.

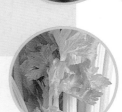

To relieve bloating
• Root vegetable soups and stews – the roots and cooking style move energy down.

To relieve poor circulation
• Miso soup with fried onion and ginger – this will strongly move energy out to the periphery of your body.
• Fried garlic rice – the rice provides strong energy and the garlic helps move it out.

Weak inside
• Pressure-cooked whole grains – moves the slow-burning energy of the grains deep inside.
• Vegetable stew or casserole with round vegetables – opens up the energy deep inside.

need to establish which pattern works best for you.

It is also beneficial to leave at least two hours between your evening meal and going to bed. During sleep, your body should be regenerating and repairing cells but when you eat, a proportion of your blood will go into aiding the digestion and absorption of foods, disrupting the regeneration and repair process. Also, your digestive system is aided by gravity and lying down with a full stomach can further slow the process.

How to eat

It is important to be physically relaxed when eating, so sit instead of standing or walking. Try to sit up straight so that your digestive system is in a good position to receive the food. If you slouch, your digestive system may become compressed, making it work harder and less open to absorbing new energy from the foods.

Avoid rushing your meal as this will strain your organs and, in the long-term, can lead to digestive complaints. Try to take your time and enjoy your meals, make the absorption of sustenance and energy a celebration. To be able to absorb the energy of the foods effectively, you should be relaxed and open. If you feel particularly tense or stressed, it would be better to wait a few minutes and make an effort to calm down before eating.

You will find it helpful to chew your foods as much as possible. This physically breaks down the food, making it easier for your digestive juices to act on the foods and ensuring better digestion.

Try to chew your food at least 30 times per mouthful. It can be hard to keep the food in your mouth, so you may need to consciously think about what you are doing and make a special effort to move the food to the front of your mouth. If you suffer from digestive or absorption problems, increase to 100 chews per mouthful.

The healing kitchen

Whenever you have the choice, choose gas on which to cook. From a practical perspective, the heat from a gas cooker is easier to control, making it easier to sauté and simmer foods. From a macrobiotic viewpoint, it is better not to cook the foods in a strong electromagnetic field as this will influence the energy and life-force of the foods you are going to eat.

Similarly, it is not a good idea to microwave foods, as this subjects them to an even more intense field, distorting their natural flow of energy. This is important because the whole point of eating the foods is to benefit from their natural life force.

Avoid pans that could introduce toxic particles or undesirable metals into your food. This applies to aluminium and non-stick cookware where the surfaces are relatively soft

 enjoy your food

Thinking about the food you eat and the ways in which you prepare it may seem like a chore, but as you become more aware of the value of good food, you may find you begin to take pleasure in the preparation.

and the materials potentially harmful. You can choose pans according to the way you want to influence the foods' energy. A heavy, cast-iron pan with a lid will contain the energy of the foods being cooked more strongly, helping to give you greater energy for inner strength. A light stainless steel pan will be better for blanching vegetables quickly, allowing the energy to be more open. A light wooden steamer encourages energy to rise.

In the same way, when using utensils choose those made from natural materials such as wood, metal, or porcelain. A wooden chopping board is preferable to plastic. Try to store your foods in a natural environment where their living energy will not be greatly disturbed.

Contraindications

When beginning a diet that is low in fats, you may start to lose the fatty deposits around your body. If those deposits also contain stored toxins they will be temporarily released back into your blood. This can cause headaches, tiredness, and extreme emotions. If this happens, it usually lasts about three days.

You may find that you suffer from diarrhea during the first few weeks. This is most likely to happen if your digestive system is not used to working with high-fiber whole foods. It may take a few weeks for your digestive system to get used to assimilating your new foods.

If you have difficulty in absorbing whole foods, you could find that you begin to lose weight and feel tired. If this happens, introduce more processed grains, such as pasta and fish, into your diet.

Over the long term, a vegan-style macrobiotic diet can lead to deficiencies in vitamins B_{12} and D (see pages 33–4). Because of the way your liver stores vitamin B_{12} this is unlikely to occur for at least a year, but you should ensure that you have adequate sources of both these vitamins. If you are concerned, make sure you include fish and seafood in your diet twice a week.

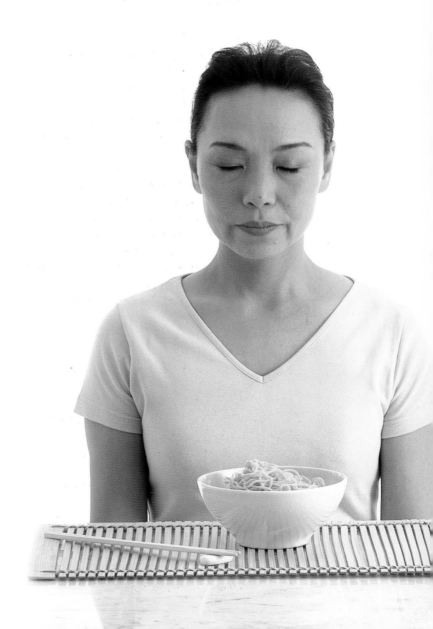

lentil soup p.126

VEGETABLES
30%

japanese rice balls p.133

GRAINS
40%

sauerkraut

PICKLE
10%

the **macrobiotic** kitchen

This chapter outlines all the various foodstuffs found in the typical macrobiotic store cupboard, where to buy them, how to store them, beneficial nutrients they contain, and how they will help you, along with tips on preparation and cooking.

steamed greens

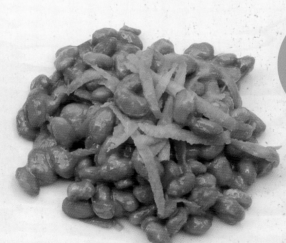

natto p.139

BEANS

20%

vegetables

It's hard not to be aware of the benefits of eating vegetables. New research highlighting particular nutrients appears regularly and many eminent studies have found that diets rich in vegetables and fruits are associated with a reduced risk of chronic diseases and many types of cancer. But, more generally, it is an accepted fact that vegetables provide essential vitamins, minerals, fiber, and other substances that are important for good all-around health.

From the macrobiotic perspective, vegetables are very important, forming 40 to 50 percent of the diet and providing infinite variety and scope for preparing nutritious and appealing meals. The vegetables eaten should be organic, or as natural as possible, locally grown and in season, as these vegetables will help you to adapt to the rhythms of each season and connect you more closely to your living environment.

the energy of vegetables

Vegetables in the macrobiotic diet are grouped into those that grow up in the air, those that spread out just under or on top of the ground, those that grow horizontally, and those that push down into the ground. Ideally, you should eat a combination of vegetables that grow up, out, and down at each meal, and some vegetables that grow horizontally each week (see pages 20–21 for examples).

How can vegetables help?

A recent study found that increasing your intake of vegetables by just one portion per day may lower the risk of heart disease by as much as 40 percent and the risk of stroke by 6 percent. Scientific evidence for the protective power of vegetables is growing fast, and one of the main recommendations, apart from incorporating at least 3–5 servings of vegetables in your daily diet, is that you should also eat a range of colors. This is because each color group provides a range of health-giving vitamins, minerals, and phytochemicals.

Phytochemicals are antioxidants, which work to protect our bodies from harmful substances called free radicals, an excess of which may predispose us to cancers and heart disease. They are found to be so beneficial that they may soon be classified as essential nutrients.

Some key phytochemicals are:
Carotenoids – powerful antioxidants that protect against cancers and heart disease.
Bioflavonoids – powerful antioxidants that stimulate the immune system. They are also anti-inflammatory and protect against cancer.
Glucosinolates – powerful detoxifiers that boost the immune system.
Phytoestrogens – reduce the risk of hormone-dependent cancers such as breast and cervical cancer.
Organosulphides – antioxidants that stimulate the immune system.

the color factor

Green vegetables, such as arugula, bok choy, broccoli, Brussels sprouts, cabbage, greens, Chinese cabbage, collard greens, kale, kohlrabi, mustard greens, radish tops, spring greens, turnip greens, and watercress, contain particularly large amounts of chlorophyll, which is a detoxifier and has anti-cancer properties

Red vegetables, such as tomatoes, sweet peppers, and radishes, are good sources of vitamins C and E, beta-carotene, and many phytochemicals, including lycopene. Lycopene is responsible for the natural red color in tomatoes and has been found to protect against heart disease and certain cancers.

Orange vegetables, such as carrots, pumpkin, rutabaga, and sweet peppers, provide flavonoids, antioxidant phytochemicals that help with the absorption of vitamin C. Pumpkin and squashes contain four times more beta-carotene than a large carrot – impressive when you consider that a single carrot provides the recommended daily intake of beta-carotene.

Yellow vegetables, such as zucchini, bean sprouts, marrow, and sweetcorn, provide carotenoids, which also help to protect against cancer and heart disease.

Purple vegetables, such as eggplant, beetroot, and red cabbage, contain good amounts of vitamin C and are rich in bioflavonoids.

Vegetable superfoods

Most vegetables contain good amounts of essential nutrients, but some are classed as "superfoods." Carrots, for example, earn their superfood title because of the beta-carotene they contain, which converts to vitamin A in the body, an essential vitamin for vision and normal growth and development.

Green leafy vegetables – such as broccoli, spinach, cabbage, kale, collard greens, bok choy, and kohlrabi – all contain beta-carotene and vitamin C in varying amounts, and scientists believe that it's the combination of these antioxidant nutrients, dietary fiber, folate, and other constituents that work together as anti-cancer agents. Spinach, Brussels sprouts, and broccoli are all important sources of folate, essential for the formation of healthy red blood cells.

The volatile oils in parsley have been shown to inhibit tumor formation, particularly in the lungs. The activity of parsley's volatile oils qualify it as a "chemoprotective" food, a food that can help neutralize particular types of carcinogens such as the benzopyrenes that are found in cigarette smoke, charcoal grill smoke, and the smoke produced by industrial incinerators.

The lily family includes garlic and onions, both of which contain sulfur

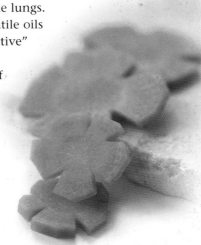

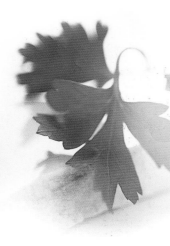

compounds, and several studies have shown that they prevent cancer and can inhibit the progression of existing cancers.

Numerous studies have also demonstrated that regular consumption of garlic lowers blood pressure and helps prevent atherosclerosis and diabetic heart disease, and reduces the risk of heart attack or stroke. According to a recent article in the journal *Preventive Medicine*, garlic also inhibits coronary artery calcification.

One reason for garlic's beneficial effects may be its ability to lessen the

antioxidants

As part of its defence mechanism the body produces substances called antioxidants, which effectively neutralize free radicals – by-products of normal metabolic processes in the body such as breathing, but also produced by environmental pollution, cigarette smoke, and radiation from the sun – before they can begin to damage cells. Antioxidants are also present in some foods, particularly as phytochemicals in fresh vegetables and fruits, and regularly eating these foods can boost your protection against free radicals.

amount of free radicals present in the bloodstream. A study at Faith University in Istanbul, found that people eating garlic daily had a greatly reduced presence of *Helicobacter pylori*, the bacteria that is responsible for most peptic ulcers. Those individuals who ate both raw and cooked garlic had lower levels than those who ate their garlic only raw or only cooked.

Shiitake mushrooms have also been studied for their anti-cancer properties. They also contain an active compound called lentinan. It is thought that lentinan is able to stimulate the immune system, strengthening its ability to fight infection and disease. Another active compound found in shiitake mushrooms, eritadenine, is known to lower cholesterol levels.

Buying and storing
Buy your vegetables fresh, organic, and in season – even better, try growing your own. Choose vegetables that are firm to the touch, have a rich color and have no wrinkled skin or yellowing leaves.

Keep vegetables in a cool, dry place. If you can, keep greens with their stalks in water, as this will preserve their nutrients and keep them fresh for longer. Try to eat the vegetables you buy within a few days, as storing them for too long also has an impact on nutrient and energy levels.

Preparation
Where possible, use the whole vegetable. Often the most nutritious part of the vegetable is found in or just below the skin, so for maximum benefit, don't peel carrots, simply wash them. Scrub tougher root vegetables with a natural bristle brush. Wash greens thoroughly with your fingers to remove any soil. You may need to cut vegetables such as leeks open to clean out all the soil.

Don't soak vegetables, as many of the water-soluble vitamins such as vitamins B and C will leach into the water. Cut vegetables into large chunks rather than smaller pieces, as the less surface area exposed to the air, the more nutrients you will preserve. Prepare vegetables just before cooking or serving, as nutrient levels begin to diminish as soon as the vegetable is cut.

To retain as many of the vitamins and nutrients as possible, cook vegetables for the minimum time necessary. For example, only steam for two minutes, blanch/boil for one minute and sauté for three minutes. If you do boil vegetables, use the minimum amount of water and save the cooking water for use in stock for soups and sauces.

Where possible, enjoy your vegetables raw. Many vegetables are great washed, chilled, and eaten plain. Cauliflower, broccoli, carrot, peppers, zucchini, and cucumber are all good candidates for vegetable snacks to be enjoyed in their natural state throughout the day.

Also, why not use dark, leafy greens in your salads? Instead of lettuce, try raw parsley, spinach, or watercress – all are tasty and full of essential vitamins and minerals.

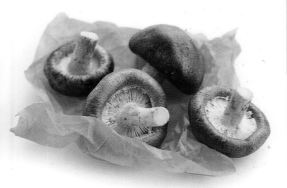

THE GOODNESS IN VEGETABLES

This chart is based on US Food and Drug Administration (FDA) figures. It shows the vitamin and mineral content of some of the most common vegetables and the percentage of daily value (DV) to which those relate. Note that organic varieties are likely to have greater concentrations of nutrients.

	100 g (raw)	DV %
Broccoli		
Vitamin C	89.2 mg	148
Vitamin K	101.6 mcg	169
Cabbage		
Vitamin C	32.2 mg	53
Vitamin K	60 mcg	100
Chinese cabbage		
Vitamin A	4468 IU	89
Vitamin C	45 mg	75
Vitamin K	35.8 mcg	59
Carrots		
Vitamin A	12036 IU	240
Vitamin K	13.2 mcg	22
Cauliflower		
Vitamin C	46.4 mg	77
Vitamin K	16 mcg	26
Swiss chard		
Vitamin A	6116 IU	122
Vitamin C	30 mg	50
Vitamin K	830 mcg	1383
Kale		
Vitamin A	15376 IU	307
Vitamin C	120 mg	200
Vitamin K	817 mcg	1361
Calcium	135 mg	13
Iron	1.7 mg	9
Potassium	447 mg	18
Copper	0.29 mg	14
Manganese	0.774 mg	38
Parsley		
Vitamin A	8424 IU	168
Vitamin C	133 mg	221
Vitamin K	1640 mcg	2733
Folate	152 mcg	38
Calcium	138 mg	13
Iron	6.2 mg	34
Potassium	554 mg	23
Watercress		
Vitamin A	4700 IU	94
Vitamin C	43 mg	71
Vitamin K	250 mcg	416
Calcium	120 mg	12

sea vegetables

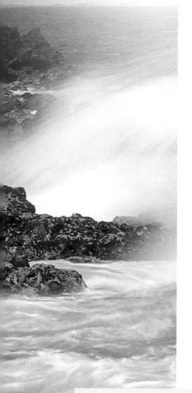

Sea vegetables are wild foods grown in the sea and harvested close to the coast. They are considered "superfoods," foods that are so nutrient-dense that you only need to consume small amounts on a regular basis to take in a wide range of health-giving vitamins and minerals.

The most popular varieties of sea vegetable are agar-agar, arame, dulse, hiziki, kelp, kombu, nori, turoru kombu, and wakame.

How can sea vegetables help?

Generally about 10 times richer in minerals than land vegetables, sea vegetables have particularly high levels of iodine, calcium, potassium, magnesium, and iron – minerals essential for good general metabolism.

They are also rich in vitamins A, B, C, D, E, and K, they are a good source of protein and the number of calories in a serving is minimal. The regular consumption of these foods in small quantities can help stabilize blood sugar levels, cleanse the intestinal tract, purify and alkalize the blood, cleanse the lymphatic system, rebalance hormones, and help to remove heavy metals from the body.

Seaweeds supply vitamin B_5, also known as pantothenic acid, which the body relies on to help the adrenal glands produce the stress hormones we need during times of psychological and physical strain. It is also useful in reducing certain allergy symptoms and beneficial in the maintenance of healthy skin, muscles, and nerves.

Another beneficial compound found in sea vegetables are the phytoestrogens lignans, which have been shown to have important anticancer functions. They are said to work by inhibiting "angiogenesis," or blood cell growth, the process through which fast-growing tumors not only gain extra nourishment, but send cancer cells out into the bloodstream to establish secondary tumors. A number of studies have also found a link between lignans and cognitive function, especially in postmenopausal women.

Seaweeds are a very good source of folate. Studies have shown that high-fiber diets rich in folate significantly reduced the risk of colon cancer. Folate is also needed to break down homocysteine, a chemical that can

the energy of sea vegetables

Sea vegetables carry with them the energy of the sea. The sea is our evolutionary mother and by eating sea vegetables you will reconnect with the most primal energy we know. It is perhaps surprising to note that sea water is remarkably similar in energy and chemical composition to blood plasma in the human body, just in a more diluted form. Taking in this energy increases our instincts to survive and reproduce. It is a life-force that makes it easier to focus on the basics of life. In macrobiotics, in addition to the health benefits listed in this section, sea vegetables are used to increase your ability to concentrate, improve your memory, and get a clearer focus on what you want in life. The energy of these plants encourages flexibility and tenacity.

directly damage blood vessel walls. High levels of this chemical are associated with a significantly increased risk of cardiovascular disease and stroke.

Sea vegetables, especially kelp, are nature's richest sources of iodine, which is important for the development of thyroid hormones. The thyroid gland adds iodine to the amino acid tyrosine to create the hormones thyroxine and tri-iodothyronine. Without sufficient iodine, you cannot synthesize these hormones, which regulate metabolism in every cell of the body and play a role in virtually all physiological functions. An iodine deficiency can have a devastating impact on your health and well-being.

Buying and storing

Buy sea vegetables in their pure form, without any additives. They are most commonly sold dried in airtight packets, although you may be able to buy them fresh in good health food shops and in some supermarkets.

Sea vegetables must be kept dry. Once you have opened the packet, you will need to keep the vegetables in a sealed container, which should be kept at room temperature in a dark cupboard.

Preparation

You can soak the sea vegetable until it becomes soft, cut it up if necessary and add it to your dish, or you can break up the sea vegetable dry and put it straight into the dish. To reduce the slippery texture of some sea vegetables, cut them up very fine. To maximize the nutrients, soak the vegetables in the minimal amount of water and add the soaking water to the dish. Also, for the same reason, cook sea vegetables for the minimum time recommended in the recipe.

In general, sea vegetables carry the taste of the sea. Hiziki has the strongest taste. If prepared on their own they would taste bland, therefore it is usual to cook sea vegetables with other ingredients and use seasonings to increase the taste. When soaked, dulse, wakame, and kombu have a slippery texture. This is noticeable when dulse or wakame are used in salads but not when they are added to soups or stews.

Contraindications

Too many sea vegetables can expose you to an excess of iodine, potentially risking hyperactive thyroid problems. Use the guide on pages 62–3 to help you use sea vegetables often in small quantities. The guide is general and assumes an average-sized adult. Reduce the amounts for children and people who are lighter in weight.

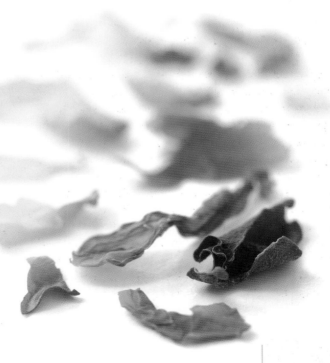

common sea vegetables and ways to use them

If you do not like the taste of sea vegetables, you can still benefit from their nutritional riches and mask their flavors by cooking them into soups and stews. This chart shows how these vegetables can be used and how much of each vegetable to use. However, do note that this guide assumes that you do not eat all the various sea vegetables at the maximum recommended levels in the long-term. If you enjoy eating all the sea vegetables, reduce my recommended amounts by about half for long-term use. Because sea vegetables are so high in nutrients, they are best eaten regularly in small amounts.

Agar-agar should be dissolved into simmering water, stirring constantly. You can use agar-agar either to thicken a liquid and drink hot, or you can let it cool down and set into an aspic or jelly. Use up to two tablespoons (dry) per week.

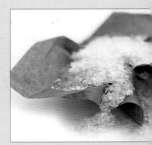

Arame needs to be marinated or cooked with strong-tasting sauces or vegetables to give it a stimulating taste. It is most commonly used in salads, with blanched vegetables or added to steamed greens. Use up to one half-cup (soaked) per week.

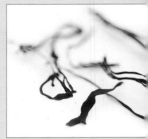

Dulse can be eaten raw but you will need to soak it for 10 minutes first. This makes it an ideal sea vegetable for salads. It can also be used in soups, stews, or blanched vegetable dishes. Use up to two tablespoons (soaked) per week.

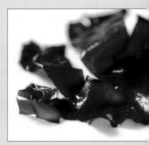

Hiziki should be soaked for 10 minutes. You can cook hiziki with stews or on its own, fried with tahini and seasoned with shoyu and roasted seeds. Use up to one half-cup (soaked) per week.

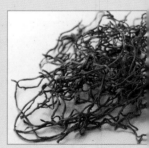

Kelp can be cooked with soups or stews. Use up to two tablespoons (soaked) per week.

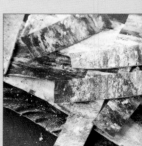

Kombu is recommended for cooking with whole grains, beans, and stews. Cooked in this way, it acts like a salty flavoring but with greatly reduced impact on your sodium levels. Use up to one 2-inch strip per day.

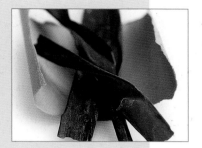

Nori is either sold in flat sheets or as flakes. The sheets – toasted or plain – can be used to make rice balls or sushi and can be torn up and added to soups or noodle dishes. The flakes can be sprinkled over grains. Use up to one half-sheet or a teaspoon of flakes per day.

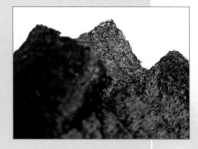

Turoru kombu is traditionally added to noodle dishes. This has a sweeter taste than the other sea vegetables. Use one tablespoon once or twice a week.

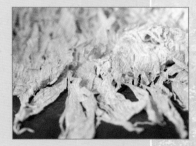

Wakame can be added to soups or used in salads. Use up to one 2-inch strip daily.

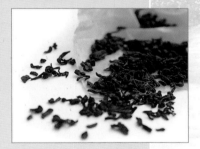

fruits

Low in fat and high in vitamins, minerals, and dietary fiber, fruits are packed with goodness and are extremely versatile.

Fruits commonly eaten in the macrobiotic diet include apples, apricots, blackberries, blueberries, grapes, melons, oranges, peaches, pears, plums, raisins, raspberries, strawberries, and tangerines.

How can fruits help?

Like vegetables, fruits are full of essential nutrients, phtyochemicals, and antioxidants. Beta-carotene, a powerful antioxidant, is the plant form of vitamin A and is present in many brightly colored fruits, such as cantaloupe and mangos, while the vitamin C – another potent antioxidant – in citrus fruits will mop up harmful free radicals in the watery parts of the body's cells.

Fruit generally has a high water content, making organic fruits a useful source of good-quality water.

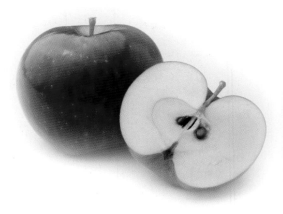

Apples are rich in flavonoids and the soluble fiber pectin, which rids the body of unwanted toxins and is thought to help lower blood cholesterol levels. Researchers in Finland found that people who ate the most apples and other flavonoid-rich foods (such as onions), had a 20 percent lower risk of heart disease. Apples are also associated with a reduced risk of cancer, asthma, and type 2 diabetes.

Apples derive almost all of their natural sweetness from fructose, a simple sugar, but one that is broken down slowly, especially when combined with the fruit's fiber, helping to keep blood sugar levels stable.

Citrus fruits and their products are a well-known source of vitamin C, minerals and dietary fiber, but they also contain an impressive list of other essential nutrients, including potassium, folic acid, calcium, thiamin, niacin, vitamin B_6, phosphorous, magnesium, and riboflavin as well as a variety of important phytochemicals.

With a similar nutritional profile to citrus fruits, berries – including

the energy of fruits

With a few exceptions, such as melons, most fruits grow in the air and, if they are not grown in greenhouses, will be subject to changing environmental conditions. This adaptable energy enables you to be more flexible and to adapt to changing situations around you. Tree fruits that grow high off the ground have an energy that can help you to feel more spiritual and make it easier to meditate.

10 fruits most rich in antioxidants

1 Wild blueberries

2 Cultivated blueberries

3 Cranberries

4 Blackberries

5 Prunes

6 Raspberries

7 Strawberries

8 Red delicious apples

9 Granny Smith apples

10 Sweet cherries

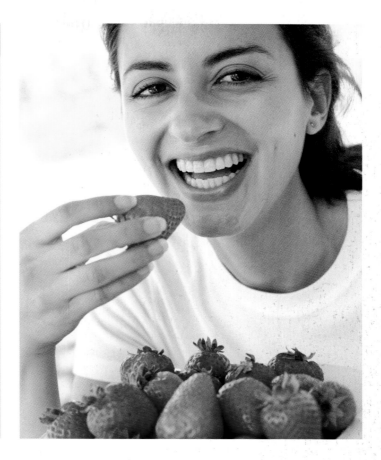

strawberries, raspberries, blueberries, blackberries, and cranberries – are highly nutritious and feature in many traditional remedies. Extracts from strawberries, raspberries, and blueberries have been shown to have anti-cancer properties. Strawberries are also said to aid digestive problems.

Darker-colored berries such as blackberries contain potent antioxidants, which may help to slow down the ageing process. Red- and blackcurrants are good sources of potassium, which regulates blood pressure. Blackcurrant skins contain an antibacterial substance and a powder made from them is used in parts of Europe to treat diarrhea.

Apart from the vitamins and minerals found in other fruits, grapes contain high levels of flavonoids, which recent research has shown is helpful in cardiovascular disease, cancer, age-related disorders, and other symptoms. Additionally, the powerful antioxidant resveratrol – called by some researchers "the fountain of youth" – is found in high

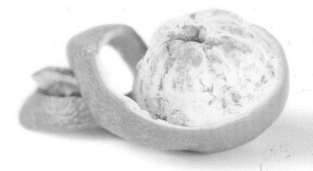

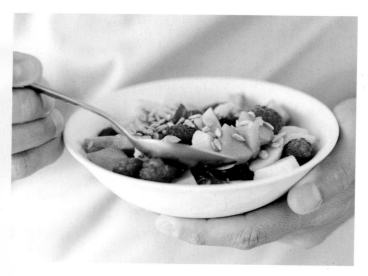

Buying and storing

Buy your fruits fresh, organic, unwaxed (if possible), and in season. Some studies have shown that the lower water content in organic fruit (and vegetables) mean that they contain a higher concentration of vitamins and minerals.

Avoid dry-looking fruits and choose those with a bright color and firm, unblemished skin. Most fruits can be stored in a cool dry place for 2–3 days but you may want to keep berries, apricots, and the like in the refrigerator. However, the longer fruit is left uneaten, the less nutrients it will contain, so do try to buy smaller amounts to eat within 2–3 days rather than stocking up for much longer.

Try to buy your fruit loose, and make sure you remove any plastic packaging before storing.

If you are going to store in the fridge, store unwashed fruit and wash just before eating. However, don't store bananas in the refrigerator as they turn black very quickly.

quantities in grapes. Essentially, resveratrol is said to activate enzymes that in turn help to slow the aging process, extending lifespan by as much as 70 percent.

Fresh apricots are high in beta-carotene and soluble fiber. They also contain calcium and potassium, both of which can help to reduce high blood pressure.

Preparation

Where possible, use the whole fruit and eat it raw. Like vegetables, most nutrients are found in or just below the fruit's skin, so for maximum benefit simply wash fruit before eating. If cooking fruit, prepare it just before you are ready to use, as nutrient levels start to diminish as soon as the fruit is cut.

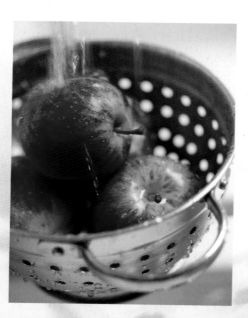

THE GOODNESS IN FRUITS

Like the chart on page 59, this chart is based on US FDA figures. Note that organic varieties are likely to have greater concentrations of nutrients.

	100g (raw)	DV %
Apple 1 medium (with skin)		
Vitamin C	6.348 mg	10
Apricot		
Vitamin A	1926 IU	38
Vitamin C	10 mg	16
Potassium	259 mg	10
Banana, 1 medium		
Vitamin C	10.266 mg	17
Vitamin B_6	0.43306 mg	21
Potassium	422.44 mg	17
Manganese	0.3186 mg	15
Blackberries		
Vitamin C	21 mg	35
Vitamin K	19.8 mcg	33
Magnesium	20 mg	5
Copper	0.165 mg	8
Manganese	0.646 mg	32
Blueberries		
Vitamin C	9.7 mg	16
Vitamin K	19.3 mcg	32
Manganese	0.336 mg	16
Cantaloupe		
Vitamin A	3382 IU	67
Vitamin C	36.7 mg	61
Potassium	267 mg	11
Raisins (seeded)		
Riboflavin	0.182 mg	10
Iron	2.59 mg	14
Potassium	825 mg	34
Copper	0.302 mg	15
Manganese	0.267 mg	13
Raspberries		
Vitamin C	26.2 mg	43
Vitamin K	7.8 mcg	13
Manganese	0.67 mg	33
Strawberries		
Vitamin C	58.8 mg	98
Manganese	0.386 mg	19
Orange juice, 1 cup		
Vitamin C	124 mg	206
Folate	74.4 mcg	18
Potassium	496 mg	20

oils

The preferred oils to use in a macrobiotic diet are olive and sesame. Olive oil is made from the crushing and then subsequent pressing of green olives; sesame oil is produced from sesame seeds. You can also occasionally use raw sunflower and safflower oil as a dressing for vegetables. Other options are small quantities of flaxseed oil used raw, and organic butter for occasional sautéing or baking.

How can oils help?

Oils such as olive oil, which are high in monounsaturated fats, lower total cholesterol and low-density lipo-proteins (LDL cholesterol – potentially harmful cholesterol) and increase the high-density lipoproteins (HDL cholesterol – "good" cholesterol).

Oils high in omega-3 fatty acids, such as flaxseed oil and fish oils, make arteries more flexible, reduce inflammation in the arteries, reduce blood clots, and even lessen the chance of fatal heart attacks. In addition, flaxseed oil may have anti-inflammatory properties that aid people with rheumatoid arthritis. As human consumption of flaxseed oil is relatively new and there may be unknown side effects, I would suggest you treat it with caution and use it only occasionally in small amounts on salads. If in doubt, eat oily fish for omega-3 fatty acids.

Sesame oil is rich in vitamin E, an antioxidant that helps lower cholesterol, and also contains magnesium, copper, calcium, iron, and vitamin B_6.

It is a little known fact that dietary fats actually aid the absorption of nutrients from fruits and vegetables. In a study published in the *American Journal of Clinical Nutrition*, it was shown that people who consumed salads with fat-free salad dressing absorbed far less of the helpful phytonutrients and vitamins from spinach, lettuce, tomatoes, and carrots than those who consumed their salads with a salad dressing containing fat.

Mono-, polyunsaturated, and saturated fat

It is easy to become confused about fat! All fats contain fatty acids, which may be saturated or unsaturated. A quick way to tell the difference is that saturated fats and oils are solid at room temperature, while unsaturated fats are liquid.

In addition to meat and dairy foods, saturated fats are found in tropical

the energy of oils

As the process of creating oils involves pressing the original food, oils carry an inward, concentrated energy. However, this is blended with a more fluid energy that encourages the energy of the oil to spread throughout your body. Good-quality oils create greater harmony within your body and make it easier for your life-force to flow into all areas of your being.

oils such as palm oil, coconut oil, and cocoa butter. Oils high in saturated fats can make your blood more sticky, place greater demands on your liver, and increase the risk of heart disease, becoming overweight, and colon cancer.

Unsaturated fats occur in two forms – polyunsaturated and mono-unsaturated – and both types are vegetable oils. Oils high in polyunsaturated fats are soy, corn, cottonseed, safflower, and sunflower oils. These contain linoleic and linolenic acids, the essential fatty acids that cannot be made by the body. When heated, however, oils rich in polyunsaturated fats become unstable and break down. This alteration can lead to the formation of free radicals – reactive molecules linked to cancer, heart disease, and aging. These oils can also negatively impact on heart health by lowering HDL (helpful) cholesterol. While we need to consume some poly-unsaturated oil to obtain the essential fatty acids not produced by the body, we should only eat them raw.

Oils high in monounsaturated fats are olive and sesame oils. These are less likely to break down in cooking and produce free radicals.

The level of saturation in an oil depends on the number of carbon and hydrogen atoms that make it up and the way these atoms are arranged. Saturated fatty acids have a full complement of hydrogen atoms – two for every carbon atom – which the body finds hard to break down. Monounsaturated fats have one pair of hydrogen atoms missing, while polyunsaturated fats have two or more pairs missing.

the components of oils

Olive oil
14% saturated fat
77% monounsaturated fat
9% polyunsaturated fat

Sesame oil
14% saturated fat
40% monounsaturated fat
46% polyunsaturated fat

Corn oil
13% saturated fat
25% monounsaturated fat
62% polyunsaturated fat

Sunflower oil
11% saturated fat
20% monounsaturated fat
69% polyunsaturated fat

Safflower oil
10% saturated fat
13% monounsaturated fat
77% polyunsaturated fat

Olive oil

In the 1960s, it was found that the people of Crete were living longer than the Japanese. Both consumed a great deal of salt but the Japanese diet was lower in fat and plant foods. Cretans lived longer because they had lower rates of stroke, stomach cancer, heart disease, and other cancers. Their high intake of monounsaturated fats, such as olive oil, was claimed to be the key difference.

People who use olive oil regularly, especially in place of other fats, have

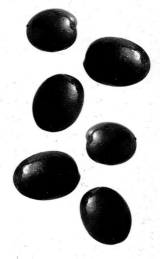

TYPES OF OLIVE OIL

Olive oil is graded on a scale that rates its level of acidity; the higher the level, the less flavorful, aromatic, and refined the oil will be. Another term that you may see on a bottle of olive oil is "cold-pressed." This means that heat was not used when mechanically processing the olives to make oil. This is essential if you want the most benefit from the oil; using heat will break down its heat-sensitive nutrients.

Extra-virgin, considered the best, comes from the first pressing of the olives and has only 1 percent maximum acidity.

Fine virgin comes from the second pressing and has a maximum acidity of 1.5 percent.

Virgin can have as much as 3 percent.

Pure also has a maximum acidity of 3 percent but undergoes some processing, such as filtering and refining, and is made from a blend of different grades.

Extra light undergoes considerable processing and only retains a very mild olive flavor.

much lower rates of heart disease, atherosclerosis, diabetes, colon cancer, and asthma. Studies in diabetic patients have shown that healthy meals that contained some olive oil had better effects on blood sugar than healthy meals that were low in fat. Extra-virgin olive oil, a mono-unsaturated fat, contains around 40 antioxidant phytochemicals, which reduce the capacity of LDL cholesterol to oxidize – oxidation is an important step in the development of atherosclerosis. Monounsaturated fat is cleared from the blood much faster than saturated fat, and this reduces the window of opportunity for the development of atherosclerosis. Olive oil and other monounsaturated fats also help to prevent the blood from becoming sticky after a fatty meal and forming dangerous clots. Olive oil has been found to assist in the avoidance of high blood pressure.

Regular use of olive oil has been associated with lower rates of asthma and rheumatoid arthritis. The monounsaturated fats in olive oil are used by the body to produce substances that are relatively anti-inflammatory. By reducing inflammation, these fats can help reduce the severity of arthritis symptoms, and may be able to reduce the severity of asthma.

Certain substances in olive oil have also been shown to be helpful for protecting the cells of the colon from cancer-causing chemicals. While most other fats are associated with an increased risk of colon cancer, olive oil is actually associated with a reduced risk of this disease.

Olive oil may be the key reason that eating a Mediterranean diet reduces breast cancer risk as oleic acid, the main monounsaturated fatty acid in olive oil, has been shown to reduce the expression of the Her-2/neu oncogene, which is associated with the aggressive growth of breast cancer tumors.

When people with high cholesterol levels removed the saturated fat from their diets and replaced it with olive oil, their total cholesterol levels dropped an average of 13.4 percent, and their LDL cholesterol levels dropped by 18 percent. According to some research, substituting olive oil, a monounsaturated fat, for saturated fat in your diet can translate into weight loss as the monounsaturated fats found in olive oil cause an increase in the breakdown of fats in fat cells (adipocytes).

The phenols in olive oil have very potent antioxidant effects and protect the body from potentially harmful free radicals.

Buying and storing

Oils will be harmed by exposure to light so always buy oils in dark glass bottles or in metal containers. Always choose a cold-pressed oil where possible, as there is less risk of damage from high temperatures. Buy small quantities of oil and replenish them regularly so that there is less risk of the oil degrading. If you buy in bulk, always pour the oil into smaller containers to store. Use extra-virgin olive oil for maximum nutrition.

Since oils can become rancid from exposure to light and heat, store them in a dark cupboard at a constant temperature. Keep the lid on to limit exposure to oxygen.

Flaxseed oil typically needs to be kept in the refrigerator; heating it destroys its omega-3 fatty acids.

Ways to use

The oils commonly used in macrobiotic cooking are all best used raw in order to experience the greatest taste and beneficial nutrients. Sesame and olive oil, however, can be used in cooking. Ideally, use them in soups, stews, and the broth for noodles, as

SESAME OIL

There are several types of sesame oil. Cold-pressed or European oil is light-colored, has a nutty flavor and a high smoke point, making it a good cooking oil. Asian sesame oil is made from toasted seeds, which gives it a darker color and more prominent taste. Middle Eastern sesame oils are aromatic, lighter in flavor than Asian oils and have a deep, golden color. They are capable of being heated to a high temperature.

the water will not exceed the relatively safe temperature of 225°F. Try to add them toward the end of cooking.

For sautéing it is important not to reuse oil and to not let the oil smoke. If you occasionally want to sauté foods at a higher temperature, it would be better to use organic butter.

Contraindications

Try to limit your use of oils that are high in polyunsaturates and saturates. Avoid cooking with any oil that is high in polyunsaturates. Excessive use of oil can put strain on your liver and make your skin overly oily.

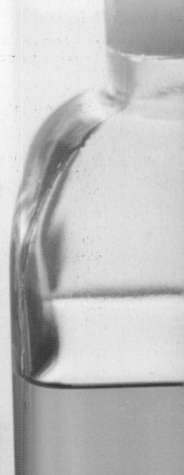

grains

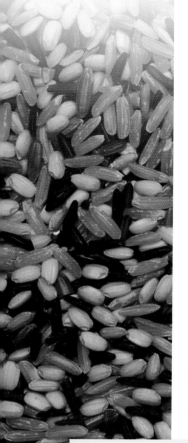

Whole grains are grains in their unprocessed, living form. The words whole grain have been used to describe processed grains that still include all their original constituents, as in whole grain flour. This is obviously not the same as processed grains, which no longer carry the same life-force and which oxidize, losing their nutrients. Whole grains in macrobiotics are brown rice, barley, whole oats, millet, wheat berries, spelt, whole rye, and corn-on-the-cob.

Whole grains are important dietary sources of antioxidants. These include vitamin E, tocotrieonols, selenium, phenolic acids, and phytic acid. These multifunctional antioxidants come in immediate-release to slow-release forms and thus are available throughout the gastrointestinal tract over a long period after being consumed.

the energy of grains

Grains carry a young energy as they are at the beginning of their evolutionary cycle, being ready to sprout and grow into new plants. When eaten, they encourage a more adventurous spirit and help you feel more enthusiastic and ready to take on new challenges. This pure life-force encourages clear thinking and a stronger sense of direction. Continual exposure to whole grain energy helps keep you youthful, open-minded, and closer to younger generations. As grains grow off the ground in the air they help you feel flexible and adaptable.

Brown rice Brown rice is the grain with the inedible husk removed but the bran layer preserved. The bran layer contains B-group vitamins, minerals, and fiber. It is an excellent source of manganese and a good source of the minerals selenium and magnesium.

When cooked, it expands to at least twice its size. Eighty percent of rice is starch; when eaten and digested, this starch is converted to glycogen in the bloodstream, providing an excellent supply of muscular energy. Rice also contains a number of useful proteins. All the grain's proteins and vitamin content is maintained during the cooking phase.

Barley Thought to be the oldest cultivated cereal, barley can be found in several different forms. Hulled barley has the husk removed but the bran is left intact, so hulled barley features a superior nutritional content compared to other forms of barley. Whole barley grain may have some or all of the bran ground off. Unground grain has the bran intact.

Barley is a wonderfully versatile cereal grain with a rich nut-like flavor. It is high in essential minerals like selenium and tryptophan. Its gluten content gives it an appealing chewy consistency. Sprouted barley is naturally high in maltose, a sugar that serves as the basis for both malt syrup sweetener and, when fermented, as an ingredient in beer and other alcoholic beverages.

Whole oats Oats are a hardy cereal grain able to withstand poor soil conditions in which other crops are unable to thrive. They gain part of their distinctive flavor from the roasting process that they undergo after being harvested and cleaned. Although oats are then hulled, this process does not strip away their bran and germ, allowing them to retain a concentrated source of fiber and nutrients. Oats are among the most nutritious of cereals, containing as much protein as bread wheat, and higher levels of fat than any other common cereal. Oats are processed to produce oatmeal of various grades.

Millet This is the general name for many similar small-grained cereals. Millet is highly nutritious, non-glutinous, and non-acid forming, so is soothing and easy to digest.

Tasty, with a mildly sweet, nut-like flavor, millet contains many beneficial nutrients and is rich in phytochemicals, including phytic acid, which is believed to lower cholesterol and phytate, which is associated with reduced cancer risk.

Millet is nearly 15 percent protein, contains high amounts of fiber, B vitamins, the essential amino acid methionine, lecithin, and vitamin E. It is particularly high in magnesium, phosphorous, iron, and potassium.

Wheat berries These are wheat kernels that have been stripped only of their inedible outer hulls. They are an excellent source of vitamins, minerals and phytochemicals. Wheat berries also contain plenty of dietary fiber.

Wheat contains more protein than rice or most other staple cereals. The germ is the vitamin- and mineral-rich embryo of the wheat and is packed with important B vitamins and the minerals zinc, magnesium, and manganese. It also has a high oil content and thus a high amount of vitamin E, a powerful antioxidant that helps protect the oil in the wheat germ from quickly becoming rancid.

Whole rye This cereal grain is available in its whole or cracked grain form or as flour or flakes. Because it is difficult to separate the germ and bran from the endosperm of rye, rye flour usually retains a large quantity of nutrients, in contrast to refined wheat flour. It is an excellent source of manganese and a good source of protein.

Corn-on-the-cob Although we often associate corn with the color yellow, it actually comes in host of different varieties that range in color from white to black and blue. Corn is a good source of many nutrients including thiamin (vitamin B_1), pantothenic acid (vitamin B_5), folate, dietary fiber, vitamin C, phosphorous, and manganese.

How can grains help?
Diabetes According to *Diabetes Care*, three or more servings of whole grains a day reduces the risk of developing

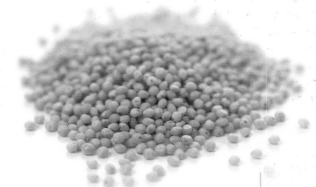

insulin resistance and metabolic syndrome, precursors of both type 2 diabetes and cardiovascular disease. Whole grains are recommended by the American Diabetes Association for diabetes prevention.

Cardiovascular disease Studies published in the *American Journal of Clinical Nutrition* suggest that barley's fiber has multiple beneficial effects on cholesterol; that eating three servings of whole grains daily will result in a 29 percent lower risk of cardiovascular disease; and that the oil in the bran of brown rice lowers LDL cholesterol by 7 percent.

Two further studies confirmed that an increased fiber intake lowered risks of cardiovascular disease. The first showed that people eating 21 grams of fiber daily reduced their risk of heart disease by 12 percent. The second showed that, for each 10 grams of fiber consumed per day, there was a 14 percent reduction in heart disease risk and a 25 percent reduction in risk of dying from heart disease.

A study published in the *British Journal of Nutrition* suggests that diets high in rice protein can help protect against atherosclerosis by increasing blood levels of nitric oxide.

Oats contain a specific type of fiber known as beta-glucan. Individuals with high cholesterol consuming one bowl of oats can lower total cholesterol by 8–23 percent. Each 1 percent drop in serum cholesterol translates to a 2 percent decrease in the risk of developing heart disease.

Whole grains are high in niacin, that can help reduce total cholesterol and LDL levels, reducing the risk of atherosclerosis. Niacin may also help prevent free radicals from oxidizing LDL, which otherwise becomes potentially harmful to blood vessel walls. Niacin can also help reduce platelets clumping together which can result in the formation of blood clots.

Cancer Research at Cornell University showed that whole grains contain many previously unrecognized phytonutrients, which explains why eating whole grains lowers the risk for colon cancer. Researchers believe that the key to whole grains' cancer-fighting potential is their wholeness. When refined, the bran and germ are removed, and although these two parts make up only 15–17 percent of the weight, they contain 83 percent of its phenolics.

Whole grains are a concentrated source of the fiber needed to minimize the amount of time cancer-causing substances spend in contact with cells in the colon, and eating more than 34 grams of fiber per day has been shown to reduce rectal cancer by up to 66 percent. As whole grains are also a good source of selenium, the risk is further reduced. Studies suggest that adequate selenium intake can reduce the incidence of cancer. Selenium has also been shown to help DNA repair and synthesis in damaged cells, to inhibit the proliferation of cancer cells, and to help the body eliminate worn out or abnormal cells.

A recent Danish study claimed that women eating the most whole grains, cabbage, and leafy vegetables were found to have significantly higher blood levels of lignans, which protect against breast and other hormone-dependent cancers. Lignans act as weak hormone-like substances, occupying the hormone receptors in the body, thus actively protecting the breast against high circulating levels of hormones such as estrogen.

Regulating body weight Two studies in the *American Journal of Clinical Nutrition* looked at the effects of whole grain consumption on weight. The first stated that women who consumed more whole grains consistently weighed less and were less likely to put on weight. A subsequent study showed that increasing the consumption of whole grains significantly protects against weight gain. For every 1½ ounce increase in whole grains consumed per day, long-term weight gain was reduced by approximately 2 pounds.

Antioxidant One cup of brown rice provides you with all your daily requirement of manganese. This trace mineral helps produce energy from protein and carbohydrates. It is also involved in the synthesis of fatty acids, maintaining a healthy nervous system, and in the production of cholesterol, which is used by the body to produce sex hormones. Manganese and copper are critical components of a very important antioxidant enzyme called superoxide dismutase, which provides protection against damage from free radicals.

Gall stones Women consuming a diet high in insoluble fiber from whole grains have a 17 percent lower risk of developing gall stones. Insoluble fiber speeds up how quickly food moves through the intestines, reduces the secretion of bile acids, increases insulin sensitivity, and lowers triglycerides (blood fats).

Intestines Barley's dietary fiber provides food for the friendly bacteria in the large intestine, which play an important protective role by crowding out disease-causing bacteria and preventing them from surviving in the intestinal tract. When these helpful bacteria ferment barley's insoluble fiber, they produce a fatty acid called butyric acid, which serves as the primary fuel for the cells of the large intestine and helps maintain a healthy colon. For irritable bowel sufferers, barley's fiber can add bulk to the stool, thereby reducing the discomfort of diarrhea or constipation.

Arthritis Copper, common in whole grains, may also be helpful in reducing the symptoms of rheumatoid arthritis. Copper is also necessary for the activity of lysyl oxidase, an enzyme involved in cross-linking collagen and elastin, both of which aid flexibility in blood vessels, bones, and joints.

Development and repair of body tissue Phosphorus in whole grains is an important component of nucleic acids, the building-blocks of the genetic code. In addition, the metabolism of lipids (fats) relies on phosphorus, and phosphorus is an essential component of lipid-containing structures such as those found in the cell membranes and the nervous system.

Mental health Whole grains are a good source of thiamine, believed to be an important nutrient in reducing the risk of senility and Alzheimer's disease.

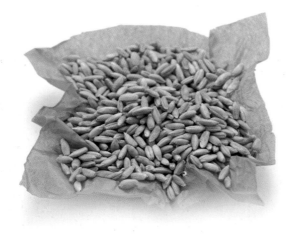

Buying and storing

It's best to buy organic from a health food store. Rice, oats, barley, millet, wheat berries, and rye are available pre-packaged as well as in bulk containers. If buying brown rice in a package, check the "use-by" date, since its natural oils will make brown rice become rancid if kept too long. For the same reason, buy oats in small quantities as its higher fat content will make it go rancid more quickly.

If buying any of these in bulk, make sure that the bins are covered and that the store has a good turnover to ensure their freshness. Whichever way you buy them, make sure that there is no sign of moisture present.

Look for corn with fresh, green husks that have not dried out. The husk should envelope the ear, not fit too loosely around it. The kernels should be plump and tightly arranged in rows. You can test for the juiciness of the corn by taking your fingernail and pressing on a kernel. Fresh corn will exude a white milky substance.

Brown rice still has an oil-rich germ, so it is more susceptible to becoming rancid. Store it in an airtight container in the refrigerator, where it will stay fresh for about six months.

Wheat berries, millet, and rye should be stored in an airtight container in a cool, dry, and dark place. They will keep for two to three months.

Store barley in a tightly covered glass container in a cool, dry place. Barley can also be stored in the refrigerator during periods of warmer weather. It will keep for two months.

Store corn in a plastic bag in the refrigerator. Do not remove its husk since this will protect its flavor. To enjoy its optimal sweetness, corn should be eaten as soon as possible.

Preparation

Pre-soak grains for at least three hours, preferably soak in the morning for use in the evening. Add a pinch of salt or a 1-inch strip of kombu for each cup of grain. Whole grains contain phytic acid, which is thought to bind with calcium, magnesium, copper, iron and zinc in the intestines, potentially blocking their absorption, but presoaking grains enables your body to better absorb all the minerals.

You can cook several cups of mixed whole grains in one pot and keep leftovers in the fridge. Mix different grains like brown rice with rye, barley, wheat berries and/or whole oats to get the broadest range of nutrients.

Contraindications

For long-term health, limit your intake of grains to a maximum of half your daily food. Too great a proportion of grains risks over-acidity and denies you other important nutrients from vegetables, beans, soy products, sea vegetables, seeds, nuts, and fermented foods.

THE GOODNESS IN GRAINS

The nutrients are based on one cup of raw grain using US FDA daily values. One cup of raw grain makes three to four cups of cooked grain, a typical daily quantity (i.e. two meals).

	1 cup (raw)	DV %		1 cup (raw)	DV %
Rice, brown			Folate	170 mcg	42
Manganese	7.11 mg	355	B_6	0.77 mg	38
Magnesium	271.70 mg	67	Riboflavin	0.58 mg	34
Thiamin	0.78 mg	52	Iron	6.02 mg	33
Phosphorus	501.60 mg	50	Zinc	3.36 mg	22
B_6	0.97 mg	48	Potassium	390 mg	16
Niacin	8.19 mg	40			
Protein	14 g	28	**Wheat, hard red spring**		
Copper	0.53 mg	26	Manganese	7.79 mg	389
Zinc	3.84 mg	25	Selenium	135.74 mcg	193
Dietary fiber	6 g	24	Dietary Fiber	23 g	92
Potassium	509.20 mg	21	Thiamin	0.97 mg	64
Iron	3.42 mg	19	Phosphorus	637.44 mg	63
			Protein	30 g	59
Barley			Magnesium	238.08 mg	59
Manganese	3.58 mg	178	Niacin	10.96 mg	54
Dietary fiber	32 g	128	Copper	0.79 mg	39
Selenium	69.37 mcg	99	Iron	6.91 mg	38
Thiamin	1.19 mg	79	Zinc	5.34 mg	35
Magnesium	244.72 mg	61	Potassium	652.90 mg	27
Phosphorus	485.76 mg	48	Folate	82.56 mcg	20
Protein	23 g	45			
Niacin	8.47 mg	42	**Corn, yellow**		
Copper	0.92 mg	45	Dietary fiber	12 g	48
Iron	6.62 mg	36	Protein	16 g	31
Zinc	5.10 mg	33	Magnesium	210.82 mg	52
			B_6	1.03 mg	51
Oats, whole grain			Thiamin	0.64 mg	42
Manganese	7.67 mg	383	Manganese	0.81 mg	40
Phosphorus	815.88 mg	81	Selenium	25.73 mcg	36
Thiamin	1.19 mg	79	Phosphorus	348.60 mg	34
Magnesium	276.12 mg	69	Niacin	6.02 mg	30
Dietary fiber	17 g	68	Copper	0.52 mg	26
Protein	26 g	52	Zinc	3.67 mg	24
Copper	0.98 mg	48	Iron	4.50 mg	24
Zinc	6.19 mg	41			
Iron	7.36 mg	40	**Rye (cooked)**		
Folate	87.36 mcg	21	Manganese	4.53 mg	226
Pantothenic acid	2.10 mcg	21	Dietary fiber	25 g	100
			Selenium	59.66 mcg	85
Millet			Phosphorus	632.06 mg	63
Manganese	3.26 mg	163	Protein	25 g	49
Copper	1.5 mg	75	Magnesium	204.49 mg	51
Dietary fiber	17 g	68	Zinc	6.30 mg	42
Phosphorus	570 mg	56	Niacin	7.22 mg	36
Magnesium	228 mg	56	Copper	0.76 mg	38
Thiamin	0.84 mg	56	Thiamin	0.53 mcg	35
Niacin	9.44 mg	47	Folate	101 mcg	25
Protein	22 g	44			

legumes

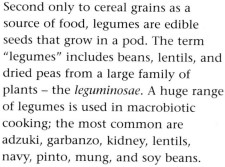

Second only to cereal grains as a source of food, legumes are edible seeds that grow in a pod. The term "legumes" includes beans, lentils, and dried peas from a large family of plants – the *leguminosae*. A huge range of legumes is used in macrobiotic cooking; the most common are adzuki, garbanzo, kidney, lentils, navy, pinto, mung, and soy beans.

Legumes generally have a nutty flavor and bring a richness to any dish they are used in. They can be cooked down to a pulp or blended to make a creamy, smooth consistency.

Adzuki beans are known in Japan as the "king of beans." They have a sweet flavor and are often used in side dishes and as a sweet. They are higher in zinc than other legumes and are also good when sprouted.

Garbanzo beans are wrinkled and irregularly shaped. They come in red, black, green, and yellow and can be bought fresh and pre-cooked in cans. Garbanzo beans have a delicious nut-like taste and a texture that is buttery, yet somewhat starchy and pasty. Very versatile, they are a noted ingredient in many Middle Eastern and Indian dishes such as hummus, falafel, and curries.

Kidney beans are dark-red in color and are shaped like the organ. They hold their shape very well during cooking and readily absorb surrounding flavors, so they are a favorite bean to use in simmered dishes such as casseroles and stews. Kidney beans that are white in color are known as cannellini beans.

Lentils are the seeds of a plant whose botanical name is *Lens ensculenta*. They can be round, oval, or heart-shaped. They are sold whole or split into halves. Lentils are classified according to whether they are large or small in size, with dozens of varieties of each being cultivated. Lentils can be green, brown, black, yellow, red, and orange.

The different types of lentils offer varying consistencies, with the brown and green ones better retaining their shape after cooking, while the others generally become soft and mushy. While the flavor differs slightly between the varieties, in general they all have a hearty, dense, nutty taste.

Lentils provide an impressive range of nutrients, including iron, zinc, folate, manganese, selenium, phosphorus, and some B vitamins. Low in fat and higher in protein than most legumes, lentils are also an excellent source of fiber. If you eat lentils with foods that are rich in vitamin C – such as tomatoes – you

the energy of legumes

Legumes carry the fresh new life-force of a seed starting out in life and are associated with growth and development. Beans and legumes tend to have a softer energy than whole grains, helping you feel more relaxed and accepting of the world you live in.

will absorb a greater amount of their iron content.

Navy beans are small, pea-sized beans that are creamy white. They are mild-flavored, dense, and smooth. These hearty beans are a good source of protein, and when combined with a whole grain such as whole wheat pasta or brown rice, provide high-quality protein comparable to that of meat or dairy foods without the high calories or saturated fat found in these foods.

Pinto beans get their name from the word *pinto*, Spanish for "painted," referring to the reddish brown speckles found on these predominantly beige beans. When cooked, their colored splotches disappear, and they become a beautiful pink color with a delightfully creamy texture. Pinto beans are a very good source of cholesterol-lowering fiber, as are most other beans. When combined with whole grains, such as rice, pinto beans provide virtually fat-free, high-quality protein. But this is far from all pinto beans have to offer. Pinto beans are an excellent source of the co-enzyme molybdenum, a very good source of folate and manganese, and a good source of protein and vitamin B_1, as well as the minerals phosphorous, iron, magnesium, potassium, and copper.

Split peas/Mung beans are small, cylindrical beans with a bright green skin and are more generally known as bean sprouts. They are actually dried peas that may be green, brown, or black with a yellow flesh. Used whole or, more commonly, split and hulled, they are sweet and creamy in texture and are often used in purées. They are very nourishing, while being relatively easy to digest – they do not generally create abdominal gas or bloating, both drawbacks of larger beans. Mung beans are a good source of protein, dietary fiber, and folate. They also contain thiamin, iron, magnesium, phosphorus, potassium, and copper.

Soy beans are found dried, fresh (also known as edamame) and in other forms (see pages 88–9.) They have a delicious, slightly nutty flavor and a very healthy nutritional profile. In terms of protein quality, soy beans are regarded as equal to animal foods. In addition to high-quality protein, soy beans also include a good deal of well-absorbed iron, magnesium, and essential omega-3 fatty acids.

Dried soy beans are generally available in pre-packaged containers as well as bulk bins. Whether purchasing soy beans in bulk or in a packaged container, make sure that there is no evidence of moisture or insect damage, and that the beans are whole and not cracked.

Canned soy beans are also available. Look for ones that do not contain extra salt, sugar, or other additives.

Edamame (fresh soy beans) should be deep green in color with firm, unbruised pods. Edamame can be

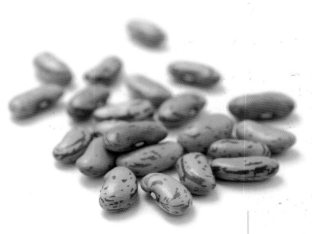

THE GOODNESS IN LEGUMES

Legumes are packed with phytochemicals and protease inhibitors that are thought to be anti-cancer agents. Although a pulse's protein is considered incomplete because it is low in the amino acid methionine, your body will transform it into a high-quality complete protein if you also eat grains, seeds, dairy, or meat during the same day. Beans are one of the best sources of soluble fiber, which can lower serum cholesterol and stabilize blood sugar levels.

   The information is for 100 g of raw beans (about one half-cup) and sufficient for one day's consumption; 100 g of dried beans will make about 300 g of cooked beans. Values are from the US FDA data and the DV percentage assume consumption of 2,000 calories per day.

	100 g (raw)	DV %		100 g (raw)	DV %
Adzuki			**Chick peas**		
Folate	622 mcg	155	Folate	557 mcg	139
Manganese	1.73 mg	86	Manganese	2.204 mg	110
Copper	1.094 mg	54	Dietary fiber	17 g	68
Dietary fiber	13 g	52	Copper	0.847 mg	42
Potassium	1254 mg	52	Protein	19 g	38
Protein	20 g	39	Phosphorus	366 mg	36
Phosphorus	381 mg	38	Potassium	875 mg	36
Zinc	5.04 mg	33	Iron	6.24 mg	34
Magnesium	127 mg	31	Thiamin	0.477 mg	31
Thiamin	0.455 mg	30	Magnesium	115 mg	28
Iron	4.98 mg	27	Vitamin B_6	0.535 mg	26
Vitamin B_6	0.351 mg	17	Zinc	3.43 mg	22
Kidney			**Lentils**		
Dietary fiber	25 g	100	Dietary fiber	31 g	124
Folate	394 mcg	98	Folate	433 mcg	108
Potassium	1406 mg	58	Manganese	1.429 mg	71
Manganese	1.021 mg	51	Protein	28 g	56
Protein	24 g	47	Iron	9.02 mg	50
Copper	0.958 mg	47	Phosphorus	454 mg	45
Iron	8.2 mg	45	Copper	0.852 mg	42
Phosphorus	407 mg	40	Potassium	905 mg	37
Thiamin	0.529 mg	35	Thiamin	0.475 mg	31
Magnesium	140 mg	35	Vitamin B_6	0.535 mg	26
Vitamin K	19 mcg	31	Magnesium	107 mg	26
			Zinc	3.61 mg	24
			Soy beans		
			Manganese	2.517 mg	125
			Folate	375 mcg	93
			Iron	15.7 mg	87
			Copper	1.658 mg	82
			Vitamin K	47 mcg	78
			Potassium	1797 mg	74
			Protein	36 g	72
			Magnesium	280 mg	70
			Phosphorus	704 mg	70
			Thiamin	0.874 mg	58
			Riboflavin	0.87 mg	51
			Dietary fiber	9 g	36
			Zinc	4.89 mg	32
			Calcium	277 mg	27
			Selenium	17.8 mcg	25

found in many supermarkets, as well as in natural foods stores and Asian markets. It is usually available in the frozen food section, although some health food stores offer pre-cooked edamame in their refrigerated display cases.

How can legumes help?

Legumes carry many of the same positive health benefits as listed in the whole grain section (see pages 72–7). Like whole grains, they are excellent sources of fiber, folate, manganese, copper, potassium, phosphorus, zinc, magnesium, thiamine, iron, and vitamin B_6. Some are also high in vitamin K, selenium, and riboflavin. Also like whole grains, legumes are found to be beneficial in terms of reducing the risk of heart disease, arthritis, and certain cancers. Their fiber helps in lowering cholesterol, their low glycemic index can help in stabilizing blood sugar levels and they will help to replenish your stores of iron.

Legumes complement whole grains in that when they are mixed together they provide a complete range of proteins.

Buying and storing

Beans can be used in soups or stews with vegetables. Soy or adzuki beans can also be cooked with grains in a pressure-cooker or heavy pot.

Buy dried organic beans from a health food store. Dried beans are generally available in pre-packaged containers as well as bulk bins. If you are buying in bulk, make sure that the bins are covered and the store has a good product turnover rate to ensure maximum freshness. Also, check there's no evidence of moisture or insect damage and that the beans are whole and not cracked.

Store dried beans in a cool, dry, and dark place where they will keep for up to 12 months. Once you have opened the packet, you will need to keep the beans in a sealed container. If you purchase beans at different times, store them separately; they may feature varying stages of dryness and therefore will require different cooking times.

Fresh soy beans (edamame) should be stored in the refrigerator and eaten within two days. Frozen edamame will keep fresh for a few months.

Preparation

First wash the legumes thoroughly, then soak overnight. Before cooking, add a 1-inch strip of kombu sea vegetable or add a pinch of sea salt toward the end of cooking for every cup of beans used.

Lentils should be cooked in the minimum amount of water to maximize their vitamin B content, or cooked as a part of a stew or soup.

Use the soaking water in your dish unless you have a tendency to bloating or gas, in which case cook the legumes for longer, two hours at least, or try cooking them in a pressure-cooker.

Contraindications

Under-cooked beans can create gas and discomfort in your abdomen.

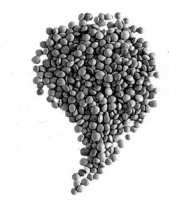

Brown lentils

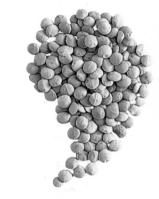

Green lentils

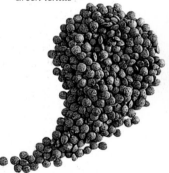

Puy lentils

nuts and seeds

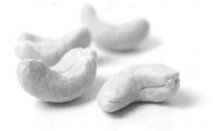

These dry, tough fruits are rich in many important nutrients. The seeds most commonly used in a macrobiotic diet are sesame, pumpkin, and sunflower seeds. The nuts are almonds, hazelnuts, walnuts, pecans, and cashews. Though often included as a nut, peanuts are really a legume.

How can nuts and seeds help?
Although nuts and seeds are high in fat, the nutrients they contain are worth having, and they are particularly useful as a source of protein. While a generous handful of nuts is 80 percent fat, it's worth remembering that a handful of peanuts contains about 7 grams of protein, almonds have 6 grams, walnuts have 4 grams and pecans have 2 grams. However, nuts are deficient in the amino acid lysine, so vegans particularly need to eat nuts on the same day as legumes and grains in order to maintain a balanced protein intake.

There is also a large amount of fiber (equivalent to two slices of wholewheat bread), magnesium, zinc (which can be elusive if you don't each red meat or seafood), and vitamin E.

Nuts and seeds are good sources of B vitamins (apart from vitamin B_{12}) and provide useful amounts of dietary fiber. The powerful antioxidant vitamin E is also found in nuts and seeds. Apart from protecting the body from the damaging effects of free radicals, vitamin E has also been shown to provide some protection against Alzheimer's disease, cancer, heart disease, and cataracts.

The essential fatty acids found in nuts and seeds have many uses in the body – energy and hemoglobin production, the diffusion of oxygen in the bloodstream, brain and tissue development, stabilizing blood sugar levels, maintaining a healthy heart and arteries, and maintaining healthy skin, to name but a few. One particular fatty acid, linoleic acid, has been shown to be effective in reducing LDL cholesterol. Recent studies have also shown that tree nuts, especially almonds and walnuts, contain fatty acids that convert to omega-3 oils in your body, which are known to decrease the risk of strokes.

The Iowa Women's Health Study reported that women who ate nuts more than twice a week trimmed their

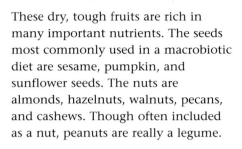

the energy of nuts and seeds

Being at the beginning of their life cycle, nuts and seeds carry a fresh, new energy. Their energy makes you feel youthful, adventurous, and enthusiastic to explore, develop, and start new things. Being whole, living foods, nuts and seeds contain a strong, clear life-force.

risk of heart problems by up to 60 percent. In another survey, participants who consumed nuts five or more times per week were half as likely to suffer heart attacks as non-nut eaters. Adding nuts to your diet one to four times a week could lessen your potential risk of heart attack by up to 25 percent.

Almonds are low in saturated fat, and most of the unsaturated fat they contain is monounsaturated – a fat that is known to be effective in lowering "bad" LDL cholesterol. About 20 shelled whole almonds provide 35 percent of your daily value for vitamin E.

Walnuts have been shown to be very beneficial in a heart-healthy diet, lowering LDL cholesterol levels and reducing the risk of coronary heart disease. One study showed a 10 percent reduction in "bad" cholesterol levels in men after eating a low-fat diet supplemented with 80 grams of walnuts. About 14 walnut halves contain all you need to meet the daily value of omega-3 fatty acids.

Peanuts contain good amounts of folic acid, a B vitamin recommended to help reduce the incidence of birth defects and lower the risk of heart disease. Twenty-five grams of roasted peanuts provides about 10 percent of the daily value of folic acid. Peanuts are also an excellent source of niacin, providing about 20 percent of the required daily value.

Seeds provide a good source of magnesium which, as many studies have demonstrated, helps reduce the severity of asthma, lowers high blood pressure and prevents migraines, as well as reducing the risk of heart attack and stroke. Magnesium prevents calcium from activating many nerve cells, keeping our blood vessels and muscles relaxed.

Seeds also contain high amounts of calcium and this has been shown to help protect colon cells from cancer-causing chemicals, reduce bone loss, reduce the incidence of migraines, and reduce PMS symptoms during the second half of the menstrual cycle.

Sesame seeds contain copper, a trace mineral that has anti-inflammatory properties that can be helpful in reducing the pain and swelling of rheumatoid arthritis. They are also a good source of iron and calcium.

In addition, sesame seeds contain two unique substances, sesamin and sesamolin, which belong to a group of special beneficial fibers called lignans, and have been shown to have a cholesterol-lowering effect in humans. Lingans are also said to prevent high blood pressure and increase vitamin E.

Sesamin has also been found to protect the liver from oxidative damage.

Pumpkin seeds also contain protein and B vitamins and provide good amounts of iron, calcium, and zinc. Because of their zinc content, many therapists recommend pumpkin seeds to men with prostate problems. Recent research has shown that the addition of pumpkin seeds to the diet compared favorably with use of the non-steroidal anti-inflammatory drug indomethacin in reducing inflammatory symptoms without the side effect of damaging

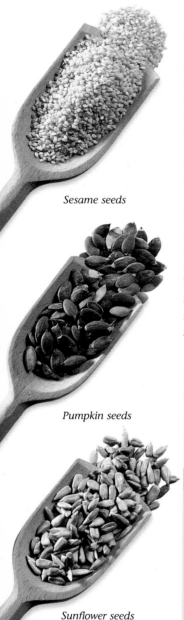

Sesame seeds

Pumpkin seeds

Sunflower seeds

fats in the linings of the joints associated with the drug.

Sunflower seeds are a good source of selenium, which has been shown to inhibit the proliferation of cancer cells, to help eliminate worn-out or abnormal cells, and aid in the process of detoxification.

Buying and storing

Nuts and seeds should be bought, shelled or unshelled, in their natural form without any additives. I would suggest you do not buy flaked nuts as they will oxidize more quickly, losing nutrients. Nuts should be crisp and blemish-free. It is best to buy nuts and seeds as you use them rather than storing them for any length of time, as they have a high fat content and can go rancid quite quickly. Nuts and seeds must be kept dry. Once you have opened the packet, keep them in a sealed container, such as a glass jar with a sealed lid. The jar can be kept at room temperature in a dark cupboard.

It is easy to roast nuts and seeds yourself, and home-roasted nuts without oils or other additives will be much more healthy.

Preparation

Avoid overcooking nuts or seeds as you may lose nutrients. As they are already high in fats, it is not necessary to cook nuts and seeds in oil. They can be used in stir-fries, stews, casseroles, and salads, as well as baked in goods such as breads and cakes.

SESAME SEEDS

A handful of sesame seeds will provide you with the following nutrients, shown as a percentage of the DV:

	DV %
Copper	74
Magnesium	32
Calcium	35
Manganese	44
Iron	29
Phosphorous	23
Vitamin B1	19
Zinc	19
Dietary fiber	17

PUMPKIN SEEDS

A handful of pumpkin seeds will provide you with the following nutrients, shown as a percentage of DV:

	DV %
Magnesium	46
Iron	29
Manganese	52
Phosphorous	40
Tryptophan	34
Copper	24
Protein	17
Zinc	17

THE GOODNESS OF NUTS

25 g serving	Energy (kcal)	Protein (g)	Fat (g)	Fiber (g)	Iron (mg)	Zinc (mg)	Vitamin E (mg)
Almonds	153	5.3	14	1.9	0.8	0.8	6.0
Brazil nuts	170	3.5	17	1.1	0.6	1.0	1.8
Cashew nuts	153	5.1	12.8	0.8	1.5	1.4	0.4
Hazelnuts	163	3.5	15.9	1.6	0.8	0.5	6.3
Peanuts, roasted	151	6.1	13.3	1.5	0.3	0.7	0.2
Walnuts	173	3.6	17.1	0.9	0.8	0.6	1.0

Lightly roast seeds in a dry pan over a low flame, stirring frequently. Roast sesame and sunflower seeds until they begin to color, then pour into a bowl. You can roast sesame seeds and grind them with a little sea salt to make gomasio, which is used as a seasoning. Roast pumpkin seeds until they pop and expand. Mix into vegetable dishes or salads or sprinkle over your grain.

You can roast nuts in a dry pan or bake in the oven. Most nuts are ready after 10 minutes in the oven at a medium setting. Their color will usually darken when they are ready.

Contraindications

Nuts can be the cause of a severe allergy with life-threatening symptoms. If there is a history of nut allergy in your family, consult your doctor before giving nuts to your child. Children under five should not be given whole nuts due to the risk of choking.

SUNFLOWER SEEDS

A handful of sunflower seeds will provide you with the following nutrients, shown as a percentage of DV:

	DV %
Vitamin E	90
Vitamin B_1	54
Manganese	36
Magnesium	32
Copper	31
Tryptophan	31
Selenium	31
Phosphorous	25
Vitamin B_5	24
Folate	20

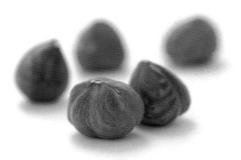

fermented foods

The fermented foods most commonly used in macrobiotics are miso, shoyu, sauerkraut, takuan/daikon pickles, dills, tempeh, natto, brown rice vinegar, umeboshi vinegar, umeboshi plums, natural live yogurt, and homemade vegetable pickles. In this section, I will focus on pickled vegetables like sauerkraut, takuan, dills, and umeboshi.

Macrobiotic pickles are made using a process called lacto-fermentation, a traditional food-processing method widely used throughout the world before the development of industrial food production. Lacto-fermentation relies on beneficial bacteria to break down sugars in the vegetables and produce lactic acid, the natural preservative that gives these pickles their aroma and sour taste. "Lacto" refers to the lactic acids that build up during fermentation and has nothing to do with dairy foods. Modern commercial pickled foods are generally not fermented but produced using methods suitable for large-scale, industrial food production using vinegar, chemical preservatives, and other additives, and are subjected to pasteurization. Unfortunately, such modern-day pickles do not offer the nourishing, living, health-promoting qualities of raw, lacto-fermented pickles.

The process of traditional pickling begins with fresh, organically grown vegetables, which naturally have lactic acid-producing bacteria on their surfaces. They are washed and mixed with a small amount of non-iodized salt. The salt draws out juices, inhibits spoilage organisms, and regulates the fermentation process. The mixture is then sealed in jars, crocks, or barrels and placed in a warm place. Over several days, the lactobacilli begin breaking down the sugars in the vegetables and producing lactic acid.

When the pickles have reached the desired sourness, they are placed in a refrigerator to stop the fermentation. In cold storage, raw, lacto-fermented pickles will remain preserved for many months.

the energy of pickles

The process of pickling is one of breaking down the components of food and transforming them using salt. In terms of energy, they have an interesting mix of the energy of concentration that comes from the salt, and the expanding energy that comes from the pickling action. In addition, pickling foods makes them easier to digest in their raw form so you can take in more of this fresh life-force. The overall effect is to encourage your energy to slowly move out from deep inside, gradually refreshing energy out to the surface.

How can pickles help?

Lacto-fermented vegetables are excellent sources of beneficial bacteria or "probiotics" and enzymes. They can be particularly high in vitamins, in some cases higher than the raw vegetable. An example of this is sauerkraut, which is higher in vitamin C than the raw cabbage from which it is made. However, because of the fermenting process, pickles tend to be high in sodium.

Pickling preserves food from decay by putrefying bacteria, while also increasing its vitamin content, enhancing your ability to assimilate nutrients, and promoting the growth of healthy flora throughout your intestines. Lacto-fermentation also breaks down phytates, which block mineral absorption. One study found significantly better absorption of iron by people eating a mix of lacto-fermented vegetables as compared to the same mix of fresh vegetables.

Choline and acetylcholine are by-products of fermentation. Choline aids in fat metabolism, lowers blood pressure and regulates blood composition. Acetylcholine is a major neurotransmitter of the body's parasympathetic nervous system, whose functions include enhancing food digestion, decreasing heart rate, lowering blood pressure, and regulating internal temperature.

The beneficial bacteria provided by fermentation serve an important antibiotic role, inhibiting the growth of harmful microbes in the intestines, while also facilitating vitamin synthesis. Antibiotics will kill off all the bacteria in your intestine – the bad and the good. But probiotic bacteria reintroduces helpful bacteria into your digestive tract, making your immune system stronger and supporting your overall digestive health.

In one recent study, Finnish researchers reported that fermenting cabbage produces compounds known as isothiocyanates, shown in laboratory studies to prevent the growth of cancer. Another study found that regular consumption of lacto-fermented vegetables positively correlated with low rates of asthma, skin problems, and autoimmune disorders.

Buying and storing

Choose unpasteurized pickles that have been pickled over a long time, otherwise they lack the beneficial bacteria and enzymes. Natural organic fermented foods are best found in health food stores. Pickles keep best when stored in the refrigerator.

Preparation

The beauty of pickles is that they go straight from the jar to your plate. Rinse off the surface salt if you want to reduce your sodium intake. Pickles are generally eaten raw with a meal. You can use them in cooking but this will destroy some of the nutrients.

soy products

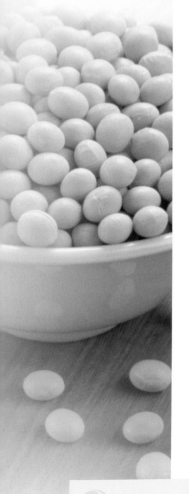

Macrobiotics makes much use of different types of traditional fermented soy products, namely tofu, tempeh, miso, shoyu, and natto. Tofu, tempeh, and natto are idea sources of protein, providing a wide range of amino acids but with little saturated fats and few calories.

To make tofu, soy beans are soaked in water then strained to extract the soy "milk." The milk is cooked with a solidifying agent and then puréed. The resulting curds are pressed into a range of textures from slightly soft to very firm.

Tempeh is made from cooked soy beans, which are cultured with a special bacteria to form a white, distinctively flavored cheese.

Miso paste is made from fermented soy beans, flour, salt, and water.

Shoyu is a Japanese soy sauce, and is lighter, sweeter, and less salty than Chinese versions.

Natto is made from molded, fermented soy beans.

All these soy products have very different tastes. Miso and shoyu taste slightly salty with an obvious fermented flavor. Tempeh has the strongest taste, being somewhat similar to bacon when fried. Tofu has the mildest taste and it is helpful to cook it with other strong-tasting vegetables or sauces. Natto is most noticeable for its slimy, sticky quality. The taste is comparable with a ripe Brie or Camembert cheese.

There has recently been an explosion in new, highly processed soy bean products. However, it's too soon to know whether these different forms still have the same benefits, and some may even be unhealthy eaten frequently over long periods of time. One recent study suggested that not only is the cancer-preventive ability of soy foods markedly reduced in highly purified soy products and supplements, but that such processed foods can stimulate the growth of pre-existing estrogen-dependent breast tumors.

the energy of soy products

Fermented soy products carry the primal energy of their simple enzymes and healthy bacteria. In terms of energy, they are lighter than the original soy beans used in soups or stews. Whereas the beans are strengthening, increase inner strength, and concentrate in the center of your torso, the fermented products move energy out a little quicker and have a stronger upward component, lifting your energy up your body.

How can soy products help?
Soy products have many beneficial nutrients and are protective against cardiovascular disorders and cancer, are useful in controlling the side effects of menopause, are high in antioxidants, and can help combat anemia and irritable bowels.

Cardiovascular disorders
A study published in the *British Journal of Nutrition* suggests that soy protein protects against

atherosclerosis by increasing blood levels of nitric oxide, a small molecule known to improve blood vessel dilation and to inhibit the damage caused by free radicals and the adhesion of white cells to the vascular wall (two important steps in the development of atherosclerotic plaques.)

One study published in the 1980s found that the sticky part of natto, commonly called "threads," were useful in dissolving blood clots.

The February 2004 issue of the *Journal of the American College of Nutrition* reported that soy products were found to significantly reduce both diastolic and systolic blood pressure and cholesterol.

Cancer

Researchers from the University of Alabama confirmed that miso, natto, shoyu, and other traditionally fermented soy bean foods contribute to a lower incidence of breast cancer. Organic compounds found in fermented soy bean-based foods may exert a chemoprotective effect.

The fiber in tempeh is able to bind to cancer-causing toxins and remove them from the body, so they can't damage colon cells. In areas of the world where soy foods are eaten regularly, rates of colon cancer – as well as some other cancers, including breast cancer – tend to be low. Another recent study suggests that colon cancer may be a hormone-responsive cancer, and that soy protein can not only help prevent its occurrence but can have a very positive effect on the number and size of tumors that do occur.

Soy foods may also reduce the risk of endometrial cancer (cancer affecting the lining of the uterus). Research conducted in Shanghai and published in the *British Medical Journal* suggests that eating soy foods may be one reason why Asian women have the lowest incidence in the world of endometrial cancer.

Soy products contain naturally occurring isoflavones, which have been linked to a lower incidence of prostate cancer.

Menopause

Soy foods like tofu can be helpful in alleviating the symptoms of menopause as it contains phytoestrogens – specifically isoflavones – which can help maintain balance, blocking out estrogen when levels rise excessively high and then filling in for estrogen when levels are low. When the production of natural estrogen drops at menopause, soy's isoflavones may provide just enough estrogenic activity to prevent or reduce uncomfortable symptoms. Trials suggest these isoflavones may also promote the reabsorption of bone and therefore inhibit postmenopausal osteoporosis. Tofu is also a good source of calcium.

One recent study suggested that soy isoflavones can help women with low bone mineral content to avoid hip fractures in their postmenopausal years.

Antioxidant and immune function

Tofu and natto are good sources of selenium, which is necessary for the proper functioning of the antioxidant system and reducing damaging free radicals in the body. Selenium also works with vitamin E in numerous vital antioxidant systems throughout the body.

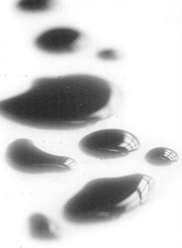

THE GOODNESS IN SOY PRODUCTS

	Nutrient Amount	DV %
Tofu, (raw) 100 g		
Tryptophan	0.14 g	43.8
Manganese	0.69 mg	34.5
Iron	6.08 mg	33.8
Protein	9.16 g	18.3
Selenium	10.09 mcg	14.4
Omega-3 fatty acids	0.36 g	14.4
Phosphorus	110.00 mg	11.0
Copper	0.22 mg	11.0
Calcium	100.00 mg	10.0
Magnesium	34.02 mg	8.5
Tempeh (cooked) 100 g		
Manganese	1.45 mg	72.5
Protein	20.63 g	41.3
Copper	0.61 mg	30.5
Phosphorus	286.91 mg	28.7
Vitamin B_2 (riboflavin)	0.40 mg	23.5
Magnesium	87.55 mg	21.9
Miso 25 g		
Sodium	1253.66 mg	52.2
Tryptophan	0.05 g	15.6
Manganese	0.30 mg	15.0
Protein	4.06 g	8.1
Zinc	1.14 mg	7.6
Copper	0.15 mg	7.5
Dietary fiber	1.86 g	7.4
Shoyu 1 tbsp		
Sodium	1005.48 mg	41.9
Tryptophan	0.03 g	9.4
Manganese	0.09 mg	4.5
Protein	1.89 g	3.8
Vitamin B_3 (niacin)	0.72 mg	3.6

Miso and natto are high in zinc. A cofactor in a wide variety of enzymatic reactions, zinc is critical to immune function and wound healing

Anemia
Natto and tofu are very good sources of iron and copper. Iron is primarily used in hemoglobin. However, without copper, iron cannot be properly utilized in red blood cells.

Irritable bowel syndrome
Tempeh's fiber may also be able to reduce the symptoms of diarrhea or constipation in sufferers of irritable bowel syndrome.

Buying and storing
Shoyu comes in a glass bottle, miso in a jar or packet, tempeh in a vacuum packed bag, tofu is kept in water within a plastic bag, and natto is stored frozen in polystyrene containers. All of these, apart from natto, are commonly available in health food stores. Natto can be found in Asian food stores. There are many types of miso, but I suggest you begin with barley miso.

Miso and shoyu should be kept in a dark cupboard, tofu and tempeh in the refrigerator, and natto in the freezer. Once opened, drain the liquid off the tofu and keep any remaining tofu covered in water in a tall glass container in the fridge.

Preparation
When preparing natto, allow plenty of time for it to defrost naturally. Natto is eaten raw and can be mixed with grated vegetables. You can use it as the filling in sushi rolls, and it is often mixed with mustard, shoyu, and a little grated radish.

Tempeh is most tasty when fried but can also be used in stews and with sauces.

When preparing tofu, squeeze any remaining liquid out of the tofu by pressing it between two cloths. This will help it to absorb more flavors from the other ingredients with which it is cooked. Tofu is very versatile and can be used in soups, stews, fried, baked, or grilled.

Add miso and shoyu toward the end of the cooking time in order to preserve their nutrients. Miso is used to season soups and flavor sauces. Shoyu can be used to season most dishes. You can use it in most situations you would use salt. Mix shoyu with equal amounts of brown rice vinegar and olive oil (if desired) to make a salad dressing.

Contraindications

Tofu and tempeh are among a small number of foods that contain oxalates. When oxalates become too concentrated in body fluids, they can crystalize and cause health problems. For this reason, individuals with existing and kidney or gall bladder problems may want to seek medical advice before eating these foods.

As a soy-based food, tempeh contains goitrogens, naturally-occurring substances that can interfere with the functioning of the thyroid gland. Individuals with thyroid problems may want to limit their consumption of tempeh. Cooking may help to deactivate the goitrogenic compounds.

THE GOODNESS IN SOY PRODUCTS

	Nutrient amount	DV %
Natto (1 cup)		
Vitamin C	22.8 mg	38
Thiamin	0.3 mg	19
Riboflavin	0.3 mg	19
Folate	14 mcg	4
Vitamin K	40.4 mcg	51
Manganese	2.7 mg	134
Iron	15.1 mg	84
Protein	31 g	62
Selenium	15.4 mcg	22
Phosphorus	305.00 mg	30
Copper	1.2 mg	84
Calcium	380.00 mg	38
Magnesium	201 mg	50
Potassium	1276 mg	36
Zinc	5.3 mg	35

Essential amino acid mg/g		% of optimal
Tryptophan	13	114
Threonine	46	135
Isoleucine	53	188
Leucine	85	129
Lysine	65	111
Methionine + Cystine	24	97
Phenylalanine + Tyrosine	84	134
Valine	57	164
Histidine	29	152

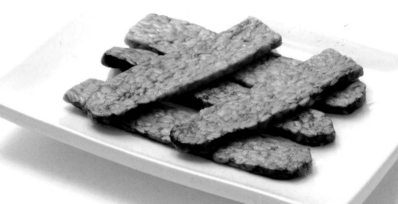

fish and seafood

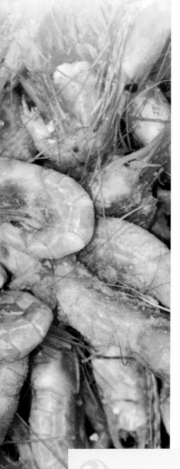

Fish and seafood (see also sea vegetables, pages 60–63) have long played an important part in healthy eating and macrobiotics. A reliable source of all amino acids, full of vitamins, minerals, and essential fatty acids, low in saturated fat but high in other beneficial fats, I recommend eating at least two portions of fish – including one portion of oily fish – per week.

How can fish and seafood help?
Although it is possible to eat a vegan-style macrobiotic diet for a while, there is a risk of deficiencies in vitamins B_{12} and D. Many fish are high in both of these and ensure a full range of other essential nutrients.

The protein from a single serving of cooked white or oily fish provides over half of the recommended daily intake of protein needed by adult women and just under half of that needed by adult men. Being very lean and low in fat, it is also ideal for helping to maintain a healthy weight.

One extremely helpful nutrient found particularly in oily fish is polyunsaturated fatty acids such as omega-3, which can help to prevent the arteries from clogging, thus minimizing the risks of heart attacks and strokes. Omega-3 also helps to improve the ratio of "good" cholesterol to "bad" cholesterol in the blood. Oily fish is also a source of vitamin D, essential for healthy bones, and vitamin A, an important vitamin for healthy eyes and growth.

Fish and seafood also contains many important minerals, including phosphorus for healthy bones and teeth; selenium, a powerful antioxidant that protects cells against free radicals; and iodine, an important component of thyroid function.

Buying and storing
It is important to buy fish as fresh as possible to fully enjoy the taste and benefit from its energy. Seek out a reliable source and find out when fresh deliveries arrive. As it can be quite difficult to prepare at home, ask your fishmonger to fillet and bone the fish for you in the store. Fresh fish should have shiny, moist skin and firm flesh. The eyes should be clear, bright, and not appear sunken. It should be unwrapped, placed on a dish and covered in clingfilm before storing in a refrigerator. Ideally, you should eat the fish the same day as you buy it.

the energy of fish and seafood

Each type of fish and seafood has a distinct energy, depending on its lifestyle. Fast-moving fish, such as salmon, sardines, and whitebait, will bring more of that quick-thinking, alert energy into your life-force, whereas relatively static seafood, such as mussels, clams, and oysters, bring a more relaxed energy. An eel will have a very feisty energy whereas shrimp, squid, or octopus imparts a gentler, calming life-force.

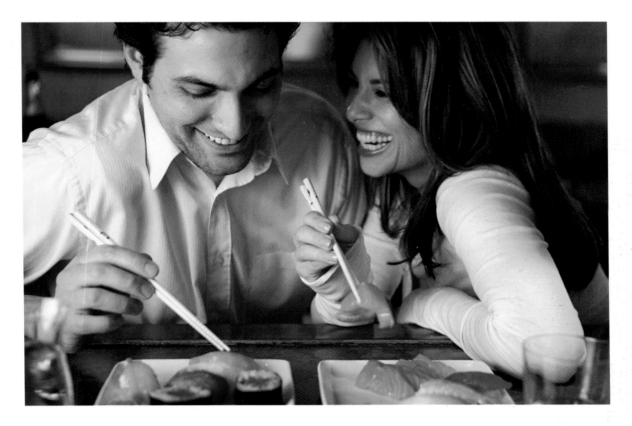

When buying shellfish, make sure that the shells are not cracked or broken. Mussel and oyster shells must be tightly shut. Crabs and shrimp should have a strong color and there should be no unpleasant smells from flesh or shell. Care must be taken when choosing shellfish, particularly oysters and any other molluscs that are traditionally eaten raw. A bad oyster – any bad seafood – can cause serious illness. Highly perishable, shellfish is best eaten immediately.

Preparation

Fish is quick and easy to cook, and any cooking method that uses no oil is preferable. Grilling under a medium heat (to prevent overcooking) and basting with lemon juice is both easy and preserves all the nutrients of the fish; poaching in water or fish stock is a great way to maintain the taste of the fish; and steaming is recommended as it keeps the fish flavorful and moist.

Contraindications

Too much fish and seafood can make you overactive and intense. It needs to be balanced out with dishes featuring plenty of lightly cooked vegetables and salads.

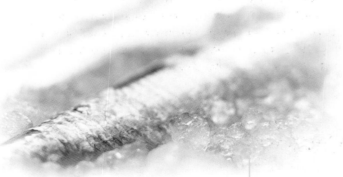

THE GOODNESS OF FISH

This chart is based on US Food and Drug Administration figures. It shows the vitamin and mineral content of some common fish and seafood and the percentage of DV to which those relate.

	100 g (raw)	DV %		100 g (raw)	DV %
Shrimp			**Mackerel (Atlantic)**		
Protein	20 g	40	Protein	19 g	37
Niacin	2.552 mg	12	Thiamin	0.176 mg	11
Vitamin B_{12}	1.16 mcg	19	Riboflavin	0.312 mg	18
Iron	2.41 mg	13	Niacin	9.08 mg	45
Phosphorus	205 mg	20	Vitamin B_6	0.399 mg	19
Copper	0.264 mg	13	Vitamin B_{12}	8.71 mcg	145
Selenium	38 mcg	54	Vitamin D	345 IU	90
			Magnesium	76 mg	19
Eel			Phosphorus	217 mg	21
Protein	18 g	36	Potassium	314 mg	13
Vitamin A	3477 IU	69	Selenium	44.1 mcg	63
Vitamin E	4 mg	13			
Thiamin	0.15 mg	10	**Salmon (wild)**		
Niacin	3.5 mg	17	Protein	20 g	39
Vitamin B_{12}	3 mcg	50	Thiamin	0.226 mg	15
Phosphorus	216 mg	21	Riboflavin	0.38 mg	22
Potassium	272 mg	11	Niacin	7.86 mg	39
Zinc	1.62 mg	10	Vitamin B_6	0.818 mg	40
			Vitamin B_{12}	3.18 mcg	53
Haddock			Vitamin D	360 IU	90
Protein	19 g	37	Phosphorus	200 mg	20
Niacin	3.803 mg	19	Potassium	490 mg	20
Vitamin B_6	0.3 mg	15	Copper	0.25 mg	12
Vitamin B_{12}	1.2 mcg	20	Selenium	36.5 mcg	52
Phosphorus	188 mg	18			
Potassium	311 mg	12	**Sardines (canned in oil)**		
Selenium	30.2 mcg	43	Protein	25 g	49
			Riboflavin	0.227 mg	13
Herring			Niacin	5.245 mg	26
Protein	18 g	35	Vitamin B_{12}	8.94 mcg	149
Riboflavin	0.233 mg	13	Vitamin D	500	140
Niacin	3.217 mg	16	Calcium	382 mg	38
Vitamin B_6	0.302 mg	15	Iron	2.92 mg	16
Vitamin B_{12}	13.67 mcg	227	Phosphorus	490 mg	49
Phosphorus	236 mg	23	Potassium	397 mg	16
Potassium	327 mg	13	Sodium	505 mg	21
Selenium	36.5 mcg	52	Selenium	52.7 mcg	75

	100 g (raw)	DV %
Tuna (bluefin)		
Protein	23 g	46
Vitamin A	2183 IU	43
Thiamin	0.241 mg	16
Riboflavin	0.251 mg	14
Niacin	8.654 mg	43
Vitamin B$_6$	0.455 mg	22
Vitamin B$_{12}$	9.43 mcg	157
Vitamin D	200 IU	50
Magnesium	50 mg	12
Phosphorus	254 mg	25
Potassium	252 mg	10
Selenium	36.5 mcg	52
Clams		
Protein	13 g	25
Vitamin C	13 mg	21
Riboflavin	0.213 mg	12
Vitamin B$_{12}$	49.44 mcg	824
Iron	13.98 mg	77
Phosphorus	169 mg	16
Potassium	314 mg	13
Copper	0.344 mg	17
Manganese	0.5 mg	25
Selenium	24.3 mcg	34
Mussels		
Protein	12 g	23
Vitamin C	8 mg	13
Thiamin	0.16 mg	10
Riboflavin	0.21 mg	12
Vitamin B$_{12}$	12 mcg	200
Folate	42 mcg	10
Iron	3.95 mg	21
Phosphorus	197 mg	19
Potassium	320 mg	13
Sodium	286 mg	11
Zinc	1.6 mg	10
Manganese	3.4 mg	170
Selenium	44.8 mcg	64

	100 g (raw)	DV %
Octopus		
Protein	15 g	29
Niacin	2.1 mg	10
Vitamin B$_6$	0.36 mg	18
Vitamin B$_{12}$	20 mcg	333
Iron	5.3 mg	29
Phosphorus	186 mg	18
Potassium	350 mg	14
Zinc	1.68 mg	11
Copper	0.435 mg	21
Selenium	44.8 mcg	64
Oysters (Eastern wild raw)		
Protein	7 g	14
Vitamin B$_{12}$	19.46 mcg	324
Iron	6.66 mg	37
Magnesium	47 mg	11
Phosphorus	135 mg	13
Zinc	90.81 mg	605
Copper	4.452 mg	222
Manganese	0.367 mg	18
Selenium	63.7 mcg	91

seasonings

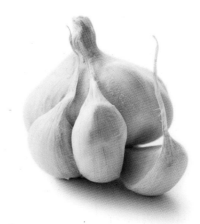

Macrobiotic seasonings include a variety of ingredients that you can add to your food while cooking or eating. They will give your meals extra taste and flavor and can subtly adjust the energy of the foods. Typical seasonings used in macrobiotics are vinegars – brown rice, ume, and apple cider; lemon, lime, fruits (such as orange and its rind) and fruit juices; parsley, basil, coriander, chives, rosemary, sage, thyme, scallions, and mint; ginger, garlic, sea salt, Japanese seven spice powder, mustard, and wasabi (Japanese horseradish); olive oil, tahini, and shiso leaves; gomasio, tekka (a mineral-rich powder made from root vegetables), umeboshi plums (pickled Japanese plums), shoyu, and miso (see pages 88–91).

How can seasonings help?

Shoyu, miso, sea salt, gomasio, tekka, shiso-sprinkle, and umeboshi plums are all sodium-rich and add more minerals to a dish. These ingredients help to contain your energy.

Ginger, garlic, Japanese seven-spice powder, mustard, and wasabi encourage your energy to move outward. These are useful for taking your deepest energy and bringing it out to the surface. Including these seasonings regularly in your diet helps to excite the general energy flow in your body, leading to stronger emotions and a greater desire to express yourself.

Herbs including parsley, basil, cilantro, chives, rosemary, sage, thyme, mint, scallions and shiso

the energy of seasonings

The vinegars, along with lemon and lime, help thin out and spread your energy. These foods, which have a cleansing effect on your life-force, complement heavy foods that contain more inward energy. They also help to keep you cool in hot weather.

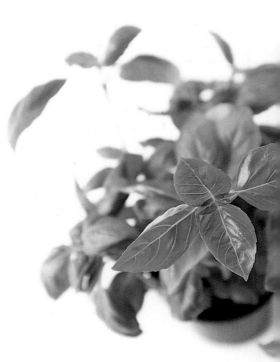

leaves will generally help refresh and stir up your energy. In general, they will move your energy up and tend to stimulate you both mentally and emotionally.

Fruits (such as orange and its rind) and fruit juices generally calm your energy while making it a little lighter. They can aid relaxation and help you feel more content.

Olive oil (and other raw oils) and tahini make it easier for your energy to relax and flow through your body freely (see also pages 68–71).

Each seasoning contains a variety of nutrients. However, as seasonings tend to be used in small amounts, on their own they will not have a significant influence on your daily intake but will provide a greater variety. This is important as some nutrients, even in very small quantities, influence the way you absorb other nutrients.

Buying and storing

Its best to buy organic seasonings from a health food store as the turnover of goods will be higher.

You can keep most seasonings in a dark, dry cupboard. Fruits, herbs, and white miso should be stored in the refrigerator in hot weather.

Contraindications

Seasonings should be used regularly in small quantities. Too much of any one seasoning risks creating imbalances in your diet. Try to use seasonings out of each group every day as they will create a balance with each other.

SAUCES AND DRESSINGS

By mixing various seasonings, you can create interesting tastes and bring a greater variety of energies into your meal. Try mixing items from different groups. Here are some of my favorites.

Olive oil and ume vinegar makes colorful, tasty dressing for vegetable dishes and salads.

Shoyu and brown rice vinegar is a dressing with a bite. Good on vegetables, salads, and sautéed foods.

Tahini, shoyu, sesame oil, and ume vinegar diluted with water makes a tasty dressing for noodles or tofu.

Gomasio, tekka, or shiso sprinkle mixed with herbs such as basil, mint, cilantro, or shiso leaves added to your grains gives more taste and a lighter feel to the dish.

Umeboshi plums rubbed over cooked corn-on-the-cob will complement the corn's sweet taste.

Lemon squeezed over fried foods adds bite and flavor. You can mix lemon juice with oil and shoyu to make a salad dressing.

Mix barley miso and white miso to make a rich sauce for cooked vegetables. You can add lemon and oil to make this into a salad dressing.

Fresh ginger (grated and squeezed) and lemon makes a stimulating, refreshing dressing for salads and fried foods.

Fine chopped or crushed garlic marinated in olive oil and shoyu will give a strong outward-moving energy to complement the inward energy of pressure-cooked grains.

Lemon, sea salt, olive oil, and apple juice make a light, refreshing, and relaxing dressing.

Squeeze orange juice onto a salad or into a bowl of porridge for a piquant and stimulating dressing.

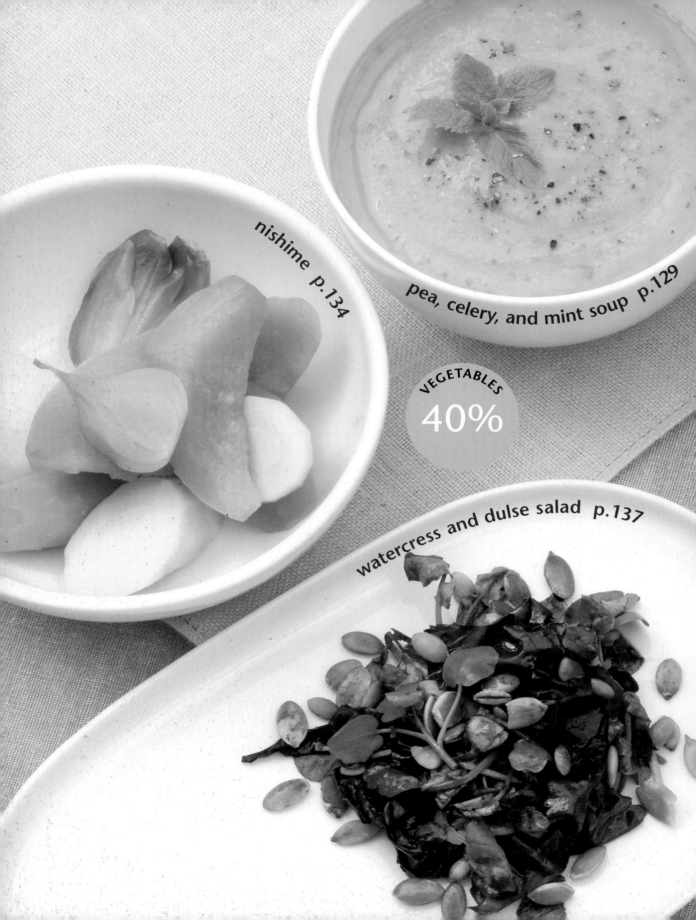

nishime p.134

pea, celery, and mint soup p.129

VEGETABLES
40%

watercress and dulse salad p.137

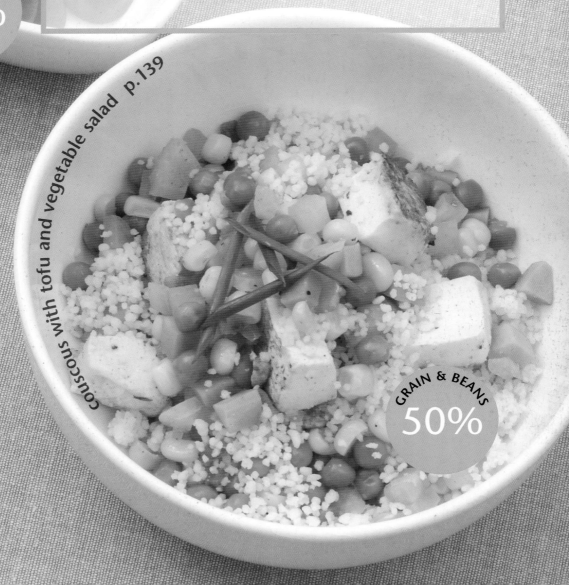

pickled radishes p.137

PICKLES

10%

macrobiotic
menus

The key to success with macrobiotics is making it work for your unique situation. Whether you want a three-day detox diet, a 10-day regenerating diet, or want to create your own macrobiotic diet for life, these pages contain all the information you need.

couscous with tofu and vegetable salad p.139

GRAIN & BEANS

50%

one-day eating plan

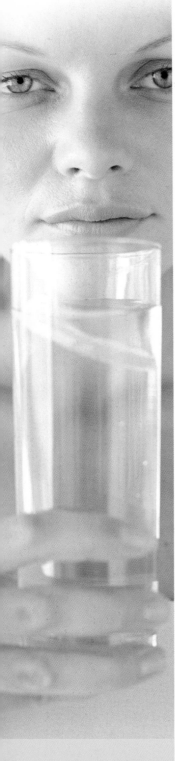

This plan is designed to reconnect you to the source of life, nature, and Mother Earth. All the ingredients are whole, living foods, full of living energy. Because these ingredients have not been processed, they have not oxidized and are still full of nutrients. This is your chance to break free of commercial, processed foods and provide your body with real foods for a day.

As these foods are best prepared fresh for each meal, it is most practical to try this over a weekend or when you have a day to yourself. To get the most out of the food, it should be eaten immediately after preparation.

Although I have recommended trying this regime for one day, you could continue to follow it for a weekend – or even a few days – as long as you include a much greater variety of whole grains and vegetables in your diet.

What will it do for me?
The benefits of eating like this for a day are physical, emotional, and spiritual. This style of eating will help contain your energy, giving you a feeling of greater inner strength. It should calm your surface energy, making it easier for you to feel emotionally relaxed.

Your liver has a chance to clean out as it rests from processing all the additives and toxins present in so much of a diet of packaged, processed, or pre-cooked foods. In fact, your whole body has the

opportunity to rid itself of some of the toxins already present while not having to cope with any further intake.

Your digestive system will benefit from a day of high fiber, which will strengthen the bowel's peristaltic action, leading to a satisfying, healthy bowel movement. The fiber also helps clean out waste that has become attached to the linings of your intestines.

As these foods are free from the sugars, additives, spices, caffeine, and stimulants that can provoke disturbed emotional feelings, you should feel calm, settled, and at peace with yourself by the end of the day.

Eating foods with so much living energy in them will increase your spiritual energy, charging up your own life-force and help you feel more alive. Even one day can be enough to give your eyes more youthful sparkle.

Contraindications
Because these suggestions contain fermented foods they will not be suitable for anyone with *Candida*. The grains contain some gluten and would therefore not be ideal for someone with a severe gluten allergy or even some forms of irritable bowel.

REVITALIZING MENUS

There are two suggested menus, one a summer version designed for hot weather and the other more wintry for cold weather. The summer style is better when you want to relax and move your energy up. The winter menu is for whenever you need to feel resilient, develop inner strength, and feel settled. The fermented foods in these menus still have an active living process occurring as the healthy bacteria and enzymes are alive. For this day, the fermented foods are miso, shoyu, vinegar, and pickles.

summer

Breakfast
- Soft brown rice (p.122)
- Parsley tea (p.155)

Lunch
- Corn-on-the-cob
- Pressed salad (p.134)

Snack
- One portion of fresh fruit (apple, pear, plum, apricot, peach, or a small bowl of cherries)

Dinner
- Pea, celery, and mint soup (p.129)
- Barley stew (without bread) (p.137)
- Steamed vegetables (p.135)
- Natto (p.139)
- Kanten with pear juice and lemon (p.146)

winter

Breakfast
- Whole oat cereal with kombu, seeds, and nuts (p.123)
- Bancha twig tea (p.154)

Lunch
- Japanese rice balls (p.132) or sushi (p.138)
- Sauerkraut

Snack
- Roasted nuts, seeds, and raisins

Dinner
- Vegetable soup with miso (p.126)
- Millet mash (p.133)
- Nishime (p.134)
- Blanched vegetables (p.135)

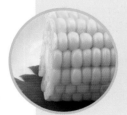
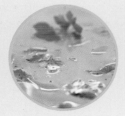
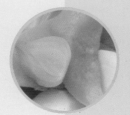
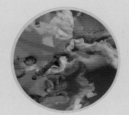
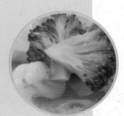

three-day detox

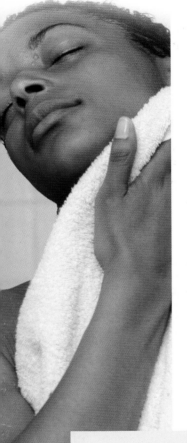

This plan will give your body the chance to cleanse itself. The foods are chosen for their ability to help your body eliminate the various toxins that it may have accumulated from the environment. This style of eating will encourage your energy to thin out and disperse, leaving more space for new energies to come into your being.

What will it do for me?
This is a cleansing detox. Cleaner energy will result in you feeling freer emotionally, as well as giving you a clearer connection to the energy around you. By the third day, you should feel more sensitive to the energy of others and find that you have a different perspective on life.

All these foods are low on the glycemic index. Over the three days, you will lose a little weight and feel more toned. Very low in fats, these foods will help your blood become less sticky, and they are also alkaline and potassium-rich to bring your body back into balance. Your skin will also benefit, looking clearer and feeling more toned and comfortable.

Contraindications
The detoxification process may bring the risk of headaches, irregular bowel movements, and disturbed emotions. This should only last two or three days. You may feel tired, slightly empty, and light-headed. Don't push yourself to complete the three days if you feel unwell. It is better to stop, broaden out your diet, and come back to this one a few weeks later.

Long, hot baths or saunas can help the cleansing process and are helpful when you wish to clean out salts. However, on this diet it is possible they could leave you feeling too weak.

JUST WHEN YOU THINK YOU CAN'T DO IT ...

At times during this detox, you may be tempted to reach for some "comfort" food. Here are some strategies to try.
• Drink more water. This will aid the release of toxins.
• Deep breathing. Sit straight and relax. Breathe in slowly over six seconds, filling first your abdomen, then your lungs. Hold for two seconds and breathe out over six seconds, pulling in your abdomen. Continue for a minute or two.
• Skin scrubbing. Take a small cotton square about the size of a baby's diaper and fold it in half and then in half again, ending up with a long strip. Hold both ends and dip the center portion into hot water. Ring out excess water, then fold the dry ends over the wet central portion of the cloth. Scrub your skin vigorously with the center portion, from head to toe, until it goes red, taking care not to burn your skin.
• Light exercise. Walking, stretching, swimming – any regular exercise over about 20 minutes that increases your pulse rate will aid the release of toxins.

CLEANSING MENUS

There are two suggested menus, one that is more relaxing and encourages your energy to feel lighter, for summer weather; the other, where your energy is replenished a little quicker, for winter weather.

summer

Breakfast
• Lemon and ginger tea (p.156) or shiitake tea (p.156)
• Miso soup (p.122) with leafy greens

Lunch
• Pressed salad (p.134)
• Sauerkraut

Snack
• One portion of fresh fruit (apple, pear, plum, apricot, peach, or a small bowl of berries)

Dinner
• Barley soup (p.126)
• Natto (p.139)
• Blanched vegetables (p.135)
• Pickles

winter

Breakfast
• Parsley tea (p.155) or shiitake tea (p.156)
• Miso soup (p.122) with root vegetables and grated ginger

Lunch
• Quickly pickled radishes (p.137)
• Watercress and dulse salad (p.137)
• Lentil soup (p.126)

Snack
• Roasted seeds

Dinner
• Barley stew (p.137)
• Chinese cabbage and sauerkraut rolls (p.134)
• Blanched vegetables (p.135)

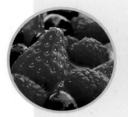 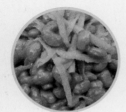 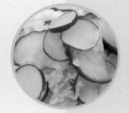 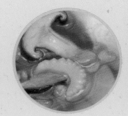 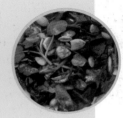

ten-day regeneration diet

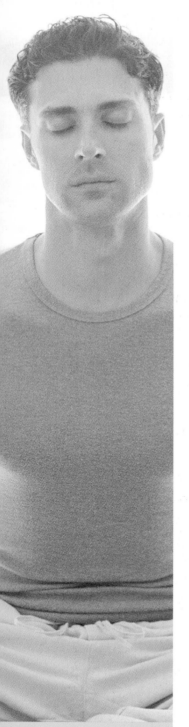

The aim of this diet is to provide you with ideal energy and the nutrients to rebuild and regenerate your body. At the end of these 10 days, you will have renewed most of your white blood cells and the energy of the foods listed on pages 106–7 will have refreshed your deepest life-force.

The 10-day program is structured so that by eating the recommended foods your old energy is gradually dispersed and thinned out, to be replaced with healthy, living energy. Many people reach the point where they release old energy but then have an uncontrollable urge to binge on unhealthy foods, bringing back in the very energy they worked so hard to get rid of. Stick with this diet, however, and you will feel much healthier.

What will it do for me?

Clearing out the old energy in your body will leave you free to experience greater mental clarity. Try this diet when you have an important decision to make, so that you can use your mind in its optimum state.

This diet is also helpful if you want to release old emotions and bring in fresher feelings. As the older, potentially stagnant energy is replaced with fresh, new living energy, you will experience a gradual lift in your own energy levels. You will feel lighter and, in most cases, happier, as though a weight has been lifted and your energy has expanded and is more free-flowing.

Taking in new energy will make it easier for you to sense the energy of

meditation

Choose a place that feels very relaxed for you and sit quietly. Breathe slowly and deeply. Every time you breathe in, imagine you are drawing energy from around you. Imagine breathing in your favorite color, sound, or feeling. As you develop your meditation, try to bring this energy into the furthest points of your body, your fingers, toes, and the top of your head.

As you breathe out, imagine your breath filling the room or space you are in. You can begin by filling in a small space around you and then slowly working up to filling a larger and larger space. Ultimately, you should be able to imagine filling the whole universe with each out-breath.

It helps to place a lit candle in front of you and stare into the candle as you meditate. Try to put all your attention into feeling each breath – the way it feels in your nostrils, mouth, throat, and lungs. Maintain this meditation, encouraging energy in and out of your body.

the world around you. Typically, you will experience a closer connection to others and gain interesting new insights into the world around you.

On a physical level, we often suffer from minor aches and pains and get so used to them that it's only when they are gone that we notice the difference. With this regeneration diet, you may find that mild headaches, abdominal discomfort, or muscle aches disappear. If you combine this with regular skin scrubs (see page 102), you will also experience a deep cleansing as the foods recommended are all low in fats.

Contraindications

If you are not used to eating whole, living foods, you may find it harder to absorb all the nutrients they provide, and consequently become deficient in some essential minerals over the longer-term. Tiredness, pale lips, or pale inner eyelids can be signs of an iron deficiency, in which case you should add more leafy greens and some fish to your diet or broaden it out to incorporate more macrobiotic healing foods (see pages 46–8).

This diet provides a narrow range of nutrition designed for a specific period – 10 days – after which it is important that you broaden your range of ingredients.

When you have been on a pure, simple macrobiotic diet there is a risk that, as you come out of it, you will experience a strong desire to binge on certain foods. To avoid this, it is helpful to go into and come out of this style of eating very gradually.

Days

1 Start with whole, living foods
to stabilize your energies

2 Cleansing foods
thin out and disperse your energy

3 Pure detox foods
release older energies

4 Simple macrobiotic eating
slow and calm your energy

5 Brown rice and barley
make your outer energy slightly deficient and ready to accept new energy

6 Vegetables
purify your energy

7 Whole grains and vegetables
bring in fresh energy

8 Whole grains, miso soup, and vegetables
strengthen your energy

9 Whole, living foods
build up your energy

10 Whole, living foods
return to full energy

DAY ONE

Breakfast
• Whole oat cereal with kombu, seeds, and nuts (p. 123)
• Lemon and ginger tea (p.156)

Lunch
• Japanese rice balls (p. 133) or corn-on-the-cob
• Pressed salad (p. 134)
• Sauerkraut

Dinner
• Miso soup (p.122)
• Brown rice (50%), barley (25%) and adzuki beans (25%) (p.132)
• Blanched salad (p.135)
• Steamed vegetables (p.135)
• Pickles
• Roasted seeds
• Fresh fruit for dessert or snack

DAY TWO

Breakfast
• Lemon and ginger tea (p.156)
• Miso soup (p.122) with leafy greens

Lunch
• Parsley tea (p.155)
• Blanched vegetables (p.135)
• Steamed vegetables (p.135)
• Pressed salad (p. 134)
• Sauerkraut

Dinner
• Brown rice (65%) and barley (35%) (p.132)

DAY THREE

Breakfast
• Lemon tea
• Miso soup (p.122)

Lunch
• Parsley tea (p.155)
• Pickled vegetables
• Steamed vegetables (p.135)
• Blanched vegetables (p.135)
• Nishime (p.134)

Dinner
• Brown rice (65%) and barley (35%) (p.132) with roasted seeds

DAY FOUR

Breakfast
• Lemon tea
• Soft rice and barley

Lunch
• Parsley tea (p.156)
• Pressed salad (p.134)
• Pickles
• Blanched vegetables (p.135)
• Steamed vegetables (p.135)

Dinner
• Brown rice (65%) and barley (35%) (p. 132)

DAY FIVE

Breakfast
• Bancha twig tea (p.154)
• Soft brown rice and barley (p.122)

Lunch
• Brown rice (65%) and barley (35%) (p.132)

Dinner
• Brown rice (65%) and barley (35%) (p.132)

DAY SIX

Breakfast
• Bancha twig tea (p.154) or green tea
• Nishime (p.134)

Lunch
• Pressed salad (p.134)
• Pickles
• Blanched vegetables (p.135)
• Steamed vegetables (p.135)

Dinner
• Nishime (p.134)
• Pressed salad (p.134)
• Pickles
• Blanched vegetables (p.135)
• Steamed vegetables (p.135)

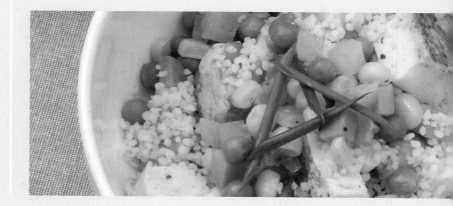

DAY SEVEN

Breakfast
• Bancha twig tea or green and brown rice tea (p.154)
• Whole oat cereal with kombu, seeds, and nuts (p.123)

Lunch
• Nishime (p.134)
• Pressed salad (p.134)
• Pickles
• Blanched vegetables (p.135)
• Steamed vegetables (p.135)

Dinner
• Brown rice (50%), whole wheat (25%) and barley (25%) (p.132) with roasted seeds

DAY EIGHT

Breakfast
• Bancha twig or green and brown rice tea (p.154)
• Whole oat cereal with kombu, seeds, and nuts (p.123)

Lunch
• Miso soup (p.122)
• Nishime (p.134)
• Pressed salad (p.134)
• Pickles
• Blanched vegetables (p.135)
• Steamed vegetables (p.135)

Dinner
• Brown rice (50%), whole wheat (25%) and barley (25%) (p.132) with roasted seeds and a sheet of nori

JUST WHEN YOU THINK YOU CAN'T DO IT ...

• Drink plenty of fluids. Try to take in plenty of liquids with this eating plan to avoid your energy becoming too contracted. Drink water or herbal teas. You can include a fresh vegetable juice in days one, two, nine, and 10.
• Keep active. Take plenty of gentle exercise over these 10 days to make it easier for your body to release old energy and make the most of the new energy that is coming in. A mixture of deep breathing, skin scrubbing, stretching, and light exercise is ideal.
• Meditate. During days five and six, try to meditate to help clear your mind. On the remaining days keep an open mind and be aware of new ideas and insights coming into your head.

DAY NINE

Breakfast
• Whole oat cereal with kombu, seeds, and nuts (p.123)
• Green and brown rice tea or bancha twig tea (p.154)

Lunch
• Japanese rice balls (p.133) or corn-on-the-cob
• Pressed salad (p.134)
• Sauerkraut

Dinner
• Miso soup (p.122)
• Brown rice (50%), barley (25%), and adzuki beans (25%) (p.132)
• Nishime (p.134)
• Blanched salad (p.135)
• Steamed vegetables (p.135)
• Roasted seeds
• Pickles
• Fresh fruit for dessert or snack

DAY TEN

Breakfast
• Whole oat cereal with kombu, seeds, and nuts (p.123)
• Green and brown rice tea or bancha twig tea (p.154)

Lunch
• Japanese rice balls (p.133) or corn-on-the-cob
• Natto (p.139) or marinated tofu steaks (p.144)
• Pressed salad (p.134)
• Sauerkraut

Dinner
• Miso soup (p.122)
• Brown rice (50%), barley (25%), and adzuki beans (25%) (p.132)
• Nishime (p.134)
• Blanched salad (p.135)
• Steamed vegetables (p.135)
• Pickles
• Roasted seeds
• Fresh fruit for dessert or snack

four-month healing diet

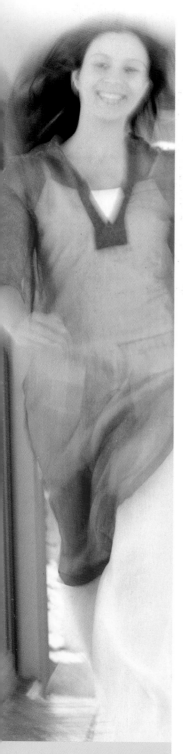

It takes around four months for your body to replace all your red blood cells, and in that time your white blood cells will have been renewed several times over. Thus, if you follow this plan for four months, all your new blood cells will have been created using the energy of your new healing foods, and these cells will transport your new living, whole food energy and nutrients to every cell in your body.

The key to making this program work is to vary your diet as much as possible. Benefiting from the wide range of ingredients and energies from all the different foods is very important, and you could miss out on several key nutrients if you try to eat too narrow a range of ingredients over a prolonged period.

What will it do for me?

The aim of this eating plan is to create the optimum environment for your body to heal itself. But you don't have to be ill to try this diet, it can be used to tone up your body and improve your general long-term health. In my opinion, you don't know how much more healthy you can feel until you try this eating plan.

This diet will help to keep your heart healthy – and I would recommend it for anyone recovering from heart disease (although you would also benefit from a regular variety of oily fish). As long as you consume adequate quantities of vitamin C and oily fish, you should also find that your cholesterol levels reduce. Eating these foods will make it easier for your body to achieve normal blood pressure levels. It can also help you combat rheumatoid arthritis and gout. Most digestive disorders begin to show an improvement, and you should find that you have regular healthy bowel movements. This kind of diet, combined with regular stretching, will also improve your flexibility.

Over the four-month period, you will also find that you reach a comfortable weight that you can maintain with ease as long as you keep physically active.

However, apart from simply "feeling better" in general, there have been countless documented cases in which individuals have defied all medical prognoses by following this diet or one very like it. It is possible that by eating this way you will contribute to your body's ability to recover from cancer.

This diet will also be of benefit to anyone suffering from diabetes as its low glycemic index foods will make it easier for your body to maintain more stable blood sugar levels.

Contraindications

One of the difficulties with eating any healing diet is to be able to tell the difference between unpleasant feelings to do with the release of toxins and the symptoms of an incorrect nutritional balance or deficiency. Although this diet is nutritionally complete, there is the unlikely possibility that your digestive

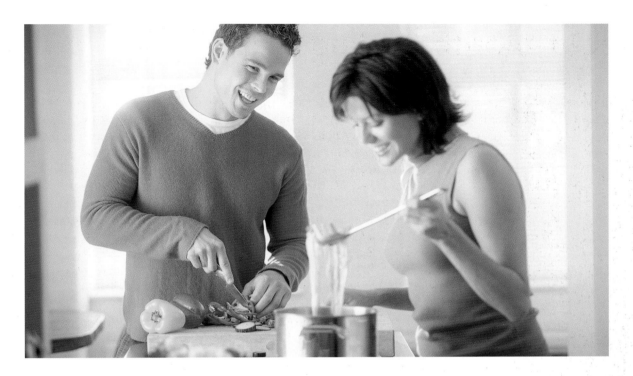

system will not absorb all the nutrients in the quantities you need and that you may favor certain foods, upsetting the natural balance of the diet.

From my experience, most symptoms of toxin release – diarrhea, headaches, flu symptoms, tiredness, skin rashes and the like – only last a few days, and anything that lasts more than a week means that you need to check you are eating a healthy variety of ingredients cooked in a range of appropriate styles. If these symptoms persist, you may need to broaden your diet out for a month and include more processed grains, fish, and raw fruit before trying this diet again.

If you have allergies to gluten, wheat, or fermented foods, you will need to adjust your style of macrobiotic eating. Initially, do not eat the food or foods that can cause you problems, and then gradually introduce them to your diet, one at a time, to see which foods you have developed greater tolerance for. You may find that cooking foods for longer than recommended in the recipes makes it easier for you to digest them. For example, if you are normally allergic to fermented foods, cooking miso for five minutes in your soup often makes it easier to tolerate.

If you decide to continue with this style of eating, do not make your food too dry and make sure that you vary the menu sufficiently or you may lose too much weight and begin to look gaunt. If this happens, it can help to use more oil in your diet. Add two teaspoons of oil per serving to soups; include some yogurt in your diet as a sauce or dip, increase the amount of fish you eat; have more processed grains and eat a dessert most days.

BREAKFAST (OPTIONAL)
Choose one of these:
• Whole oat cereal with kombu, seeds, and nuts (p.123), season with ½ tsp of gomasio, tekka, or shiso powder
• Miso soup (p.122)
• Soft-grain, using leftover brown rice and another grain (oats, wheat, rye) sometimes with beans (p.122)
• Fried mochi savory (p. 123) and vegetables

Choose a tea:
• Lemon tea
• Bancha twig tea (p.154)
• Green and brown rice tea (p.154)
• Mint tea (p.156)

MORNING SNACK (OPTIONAL)
• Roasted seeds
• Steamed bread with tahini or hummus (p.125)

LUNCH
Choose one of these:
• Japanese rice balls (p.133)
• Brown rice and whole grains (p. 132)
• Corn-on-the-cob
• Millet mash (p.133)
• Garlic rice (p.133)
• Couscous salad (p.139)
• Noodles (p.142)

Choose two or three of these:
• Blanched vegetables (p.135)
• Steamed vegetables (p.135)
• Chinese cabbage and sauerkraut rolls (p.134)
• Pressed salad (p.134)
• Natto (p.139)
• Marinated tofu steak (p.144)
• Pickles
• Sauerkraut

AFTERNOON SNACK (OPTIONAL)
Choose one of these:
• Fresh fruit one to four times a week
• Roasted seeds and nuts

Choose a tea:
• Bancha twig tea (p.154)
• Green and brown rice tea (p.154)
• Mint tea (p.156)
• Camomile tea
• Parsley tea (p.155)
• Lemon and ginger tea (p.156)
• Sweet vegetable tea (p.154)

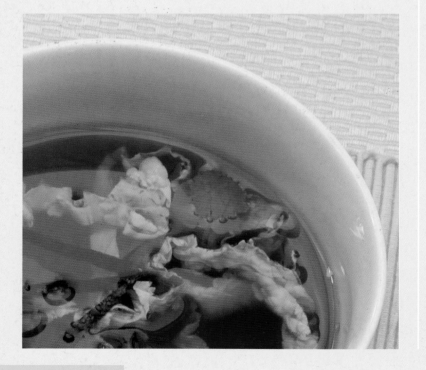

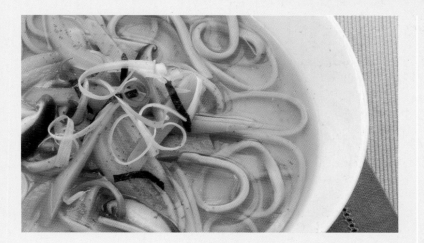

DINNER

Choose one of these, and once or twice a week add fish or shellfish to your soup:
• Vegetable soup with miso (p.126)
• Lentil soup (p.126)
• Barley soup (p.126)
• Shoyu soup with carrot and radish (p.128)
• Sweet millet soup (p.128)
• Clear cauliflower soup (p.128)
• Cucumber and ginger soup (p.129)
• Pea, celery, and mint soup (p.129)
• Carrot soup (p.131)
• Bean and vegetable soup (p.130–31)

Choose one of these:
• Brown rice (50%), barley, whole wheat, whole rye, or whole oats (25%) and adzuki beans or roasted black soy beans (25%) (p.132)
• Millet mash (p.133)
• Garlic rice (p.133)
• Barley stew (p.137)
• Sushi (p.138)
• Couscous salad (p.139)
• Nabe (p.140)
• Japanese rice balls (p.133)
• Emerald eye stew (p.138–9)

Choose three or four of these:
• Blanched salad (p.135)
• Steamed greens
• Pressed salad (p.134)
• Nishime (p.134)
• Kinpira (p.135)
• Adzuki bean and root vegetable stew (p.134)
• Pickles
• Roasted seeds

Choose one of these two to four times a week:
• Nutty rice pudding (p.146)
• Stewed fruit (p.149)
• Kanten with pear juice and lemon (p.146)
• Hunza apricots with vanilla (p.146)

Choose a tea:
• Bancha twig tea (p.154)
• Green and brown rice tea (p.154)
• Camomile tea

how long can I go on?

You can continue this eating plan for longer than four months as long as you feel good and maintain the variety. It is important to keep reviewing your health so that you can detect any signs of deficiency and broaden out your diet. Many people who use macrobiotics to recover from serious health problems continue with this style of eating for several years.

shortcuts to healthy eating

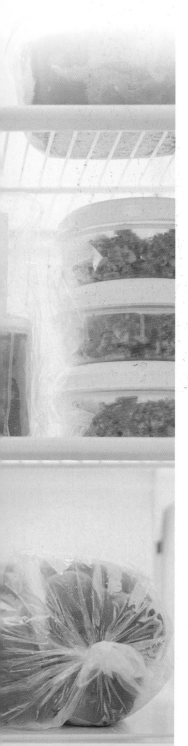

Macrobiotics is all about living the big life, and spending too much time in the kitchen does not allow you to get out and make the most of yourself. It is important that you are able to practice macrobiotics in a way that gives you the right balance between eating homemade, healthy foods and having time to enjoy your good health and develop yourself.

When I started eating a macrobiotic diet, I would typically spend at least an hour cooking a meal. Since then, I have learned how to organize my kitchen more efficiently. I prepare all the dishes that take longer to cook once every three days, "batch cooking" a sufficient quantity so that I have plenty to last a few days, leaving the remaining days' dishes quick and easy to prepare.

Planning ahead
When you start practicing macrobiotics, it will help if you plan your menus so that you have the soaked or cooked ingredients ready for certain dishes or meals. For example, if you want whole oat cereal in the morning, you will need to start cooking the oats the night before; similarly, soaking grains or beans before you go to bed means that everything is ready for you to cook the following day; cooking extra brown rice and barley in the evening will mean you have leftovers to make cereal in the morning or to sauté for lunch. A little thought beforehand can save you time and ensure all your meals are healthy and nutritious.

The essential store cupboard
When you want to eat more healthily, what you keep in your refrigerator and cupboards is of the greatest importance. Always keep a good stock of healthy foods, that way you can quickly create a healthy meal rather than be tempted to reach for a less healthy snack. The way I make this work is to always have a bowl of cooked whole grains, some cooked beans, a nishime dish, and pot of soup in my fridge so that all I need to do is heat them up.

In addition, I keep all the ingredients to make quick 10-minute meals (see pages 114–15), so that when I come home feeling hungry, I know that within 10 minutes I'll be eating a healthy macrobiotic meal.

Every third day
People tend to think that eating a macrobiotic diet will tie them to the kitchen for hours on end day after day. However, with a little planning you can enjoy whole, living foods every day but only spend more than

planning

If you can organize your schedule so that you can do a "big cook" on two nights of the week, you are guaranteed to have healthy, whole, nutritious food available to you whenever you need it.

20 minutes in the kitchen every third day, when you may need to spend around 1½ hours preparing everything for several days ahead.

You may find it easier to allocate certain times during the week for preparation. This way you can organize your timetable and build up a routine. For example, soak beans and grains and cook your cereal on Monday and Thursday evenings. It only takes 10 or 15 minutes and, as the cereal cooks, you can be relaxing or getting ready for bed.

On my "big" cooking days, I prepare a large pot of whole grains. If I don't include beans with the grains, I cook a bean stew or soup. I also prepare some vegetables that take longer to cook, such as a stew or nishime. You will need to estimate how much you need to cook to last you the required time. As a rough guide, depending on appetites, four cups of whole grains will make enough for four people to eat three main meals.

Storing and reheating cooked food
Cooked foods should always be stored in the refrigerator. It is very important only to heat up the food you are going to eat – rather than reheating all the food – as constant cooling and reheating can increase the growth of harmful bacteria and will shorten the life and destroy the energy of the food.

You can take any leftover grains and sauté them, steam them, cook them into a soup, or boil them into a soft porridge to make them more interesting. To make these meals complete, I would add light, fresh dishes such as a pressed salad, or blanched or steamed vegetables.

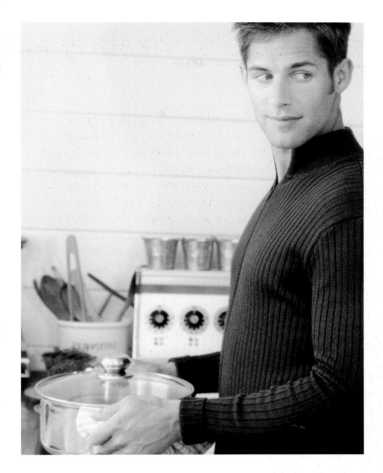

On other days, I will use millet or corn-on-the-cob if I want a quick-cooking whole grain, or mochi, noodles, or pasta if I want a processed grain. If I have run out of pre-cooked dishes, I will lightly boil or steam vegetables to go with the grain. For extra richness, I might fry some tofu.

It may seem that you have a great deal to think about and organize in order to follow a macrobiotic diet but don't be daunted. Once you are familiar with these delicious meals, you will find they are very quick and easy to prepare.

ten-minute meals

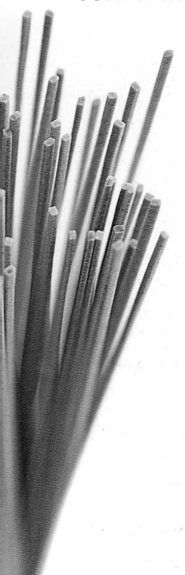

Although "convenience" isn't a word often used in books on healthy eating, it is important that you are able to prepare quick, healthy macrobiotic meals when you need them, so that you never feel that you can't improve your health because you don't have enough time. The fact is that it's often just as quick and easy to make a healthy meal as a less healthy one, it just requires a little time to become familiar with the ingredients and learn how to prepare them.

When time's at a premium

There are now many readily available ingredients that will enable you to make a healthy macrobiotic meal quickly. Mochi, tofu, natto, tempeh, seiten, vegetable, bean or grain burgers, natural pesto sauces, natural sauerkraut, good-quality breads, hummus, and tahini can all be bought ready made and need very little further preparation for a wholesome meal.

However, there are some foods – such as miso soup, whole grains, and noodle sauces – that are always much better when prepared from scratch. The instant varieties of miso, for example, never seem to have the true taste, and certainly don't contain the levels of nutrients or the living energy of home-made miso soup.

The recipes starting on page 122 all show the time it takes to prepare them, so when you are in a hurry, scan through the recipes looking for those that will be quick to make.

reheating foods

When reheating foods, only heat the amount you are going to eat, and make sure it is heated all the way through. Failure to do this can result in the growth of potentially harmful bacteria. The food should be reheated so that it exceeds a temperature of 160°F. This temperature is too high for the bacteria to survive.

Stir thick soups so that all the liquid reaches boiling point; when sautéing leftover grains, sauté a thin layer and turn frequently; to steam leftovers, put small amounts in the steamer and break them up, if necessary, so that the steam can reach all parts of the food; when boiling leftovers, allow sufficient time for the heat to reach the center of the foods. The larger the food being reheated, the longer it will take.

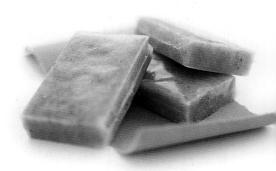

MACROBIOTICS IN A HURRY

Here are some examples of quick macrobiotic meals that you can make without any pre-cooked foods.

BREAKFAST
• Miso soup (p.122)
• Fried mochi savory or with syrup (p.123)
• Sourdough bread with hummus and sauerkraut (p.125)
• Blanched vegetables (p.135)
• Organic muesli with rice, oat, or nut milk

LUNCH OR DINNER
• Vegetable soup with miso (p.126)

Choose one of the following:
• Corn-on-the-cob
• Couscous with tofu and vegetable salad (p.139)
• Polenta mash (p.145)
• Mediterranean pasta (p.145)
• Nabe (p.140)
• Fried mochi (p.123)
• Fried grain, bean, or vegetable burger
(In the case of the couscous, tofu and vegetable salad, and nabe, they are meals in themselves and do not need any other accompaniments.)

Choose one of the following:
• Fried tofu (p.144)
• Fried tempeh
• Seitan dish (p.142)
• Natto (p.139)

Choose two of the following:
• Pressed salad (p.134)
• Chinese cabbage and sauerkraut rolls (p.134)
• Blanched vegetables (p.135)
• Watercress and dulse salad (p.137)

If you are following the shortcuts principle (see pages 112–13), you may already have pre-cooked foods available and will be able to make these meals very quickly.

BREAKFAST
• Boil leftover whole grains into a cereal
• Heat up any leftover whole oat cereal

LUNCH OR DINNER
• Heat up any leftover soup

Choose one of the following:
• Add water to your leftover millet mash and heat through
• Steam or fry leftover grains, or make sushi
• Garlic rice (p.133) or deep-fried rice balls (p.141) using leftover brown rice
• Soba spice (p.141) using leftover noodles

Choose one of the following:
• Bean stew
• Adzuki bean and root vegetable stew (p.134)
• Nishime (p.134)

Make one or two of the following for freshness:
• Pressed salad (p.134)
• Chinese cabbage and sauerkraut rolls (p.134)
• Blanched vegetables (p.135)
• Watercress and dulse salad (p.137)
• Sauerkraut or pickled vegetables
• Steamed vegetables (p.135)
• Roast seeds and add to the dishes as appropriate

eating out

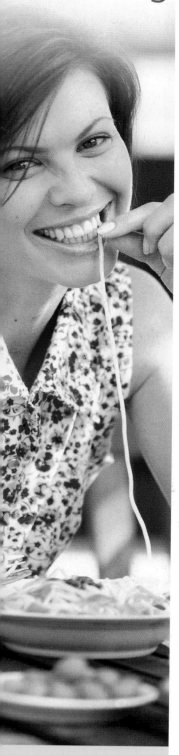

There is so much more choice when eating out now, that it's much easier to find healthy foods, even on the most complex menu. You should find that you can eat healthily wherever you are: most areas have somewhere where you can enjoy a pasta dish with a simple sauce and a salad.

Talk to your waiter

If you can find nothing on the menu that appeals to you, try asking for your choice of pasta and salad. Because so many people suffer from allergies, restaurants are much more accommodating to special diets, so if you are in the process of healing, ask if they will make a special dish for you – obviously, the simpler the better. For example, ask for pasta with garlic and olive oil, plain blanched broccoli or carrots, and a green salad.

If you do go for something on the menu and feel in doubt about the ingredients used, ask your waiter to describe different dishes to you so you know what to expect, and ask for any sauces or dressing to be served separately. If you are lucky enough to find an organic restaurant, you can be assured of better-quality ingredients.

Hidden ingredients

Apart from any hidden sauces, oils, salts, and any additives used are all areas for concern. For example, when deep-frying foods, most vegetable oils become unstable at high temperatures, ultimately releasing more toxic free radicals into the body. This is made worse when restaurants use cheap blends of oils, increasing the risk of oxidation, which in turn can accelerate the aging process.

Obviously, as you consume relatively high amounts of oil when eating deep-fried foods such as french fries, the risks also become greater. It's always advisable to check with the chef, but personally, I tend to avoid fried or oily foods when eating out.

Some chefs will mask poor quality ingredients by adding excessive salt and, following a macrobiotic diet, you could consume several days' worth of salt in one meal at a restaurant. Be aware of any cravings you experience after a restaurant meal (see pages 40–41) and make a note of them, so that you can search out other restaurants that have a more health-conscious chef.

Currently, restaurants do not have to inform customers about the use of genetically modified (GM) or irradiated ingredients, but ask the staff whether they know. Eventually, public interest will persuade restaurants to reconsider these ingredients and adopt a healthier policy.

MSG is often used in Chinese restaurants. You may be able to pre-order dishes without MSG or there may be certain dishes that are free from MSG.

If you do not wish to eat meat, ask about soup stocks as these may contain animal fats.

FOODS TO LOOK OUT FOR

When eating out, our favorite restaurants are Japanese, Italian, and Indian, although I also enjoy Greek, French, and Chinese foods.

Pasta with pesto, vegetable, or seafood sauces make a filling, complete meal.

Vegetable soup with a good-quality bread can be very satisfying.

Salads are a good healthy choice, and the wide range of ingredients to choose from makes them even more appealing. Don't be afraid to design your own mixed salad.

Vegetable dishes are often a disappointment. Try asking for the vegetables to be cooked *al dente* without butter if you want that fresh, clean taste.

Pita with hummus, tahini, falafel, and salad is a great macrobiotic fast-food although it will probably be cooked in poor-quality oil.

Noodles in a hot broth is a satisfying meal, but check to see if it contains MSG. The sauce can be very salty.

Sushi is a popular and clean way to eat fish. The white rice will often have some sugar in it. If you want to avoid the rice, ask for sashimi.

Fish and seafood dishes are highly nutritious. Fish soups tend to be particularly high in nutrients. With good, fresh fish there's little need to dress it up and coat it with rich sauces, so go for the most "unadulterated" fish dish you can see on the menu, such as poached white fish served with lemon.

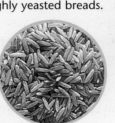

Lentil and vegetable curries are enjoyable vegetarian dishes. Sometimes the chef will add a lot of oil; however, because the boiling temperature will not exceed 225°F there is less risk of the oil breaking down.

Basmati rice is more nutritious and has a lower GI than white rice.

Nan bread can be very satisfying and less bloating than highly yeasted breads.

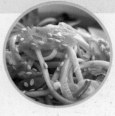

a macrobiotic diet for life

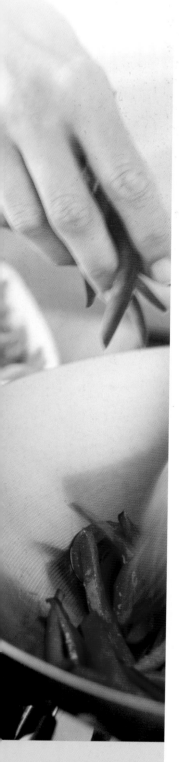

Having read this book so far you should now be in a good position to design your own macrobiotic diet. This is something that is individual to you – I cannot prescribe what your diet should consist of, only guide you in your choices. Use the six steps in the box below to create your own macrobiotic diet. As time goes by and you change, your needs will also alter, so take time to revise and update your macrobiotic practice as necessary. You may find it useful to write down your intentions so you have something to refer to.

Macrobiotics in a typical week

The best way to explain how I use macrobiotics is to describe the kind of macrobiotic diet my family eats.

We made the decision to pay the extra for organic ingredients many years ago.

We try to have a vegetable soup daily, often including wakame, kombu, or dulse and seasoned with miso. In a typical week at home, we eat whole grains at more than half

our meals. More than a half of our food is made up of fresh vegetables. We eat soups or stews with beans about twice a week. In addition, I might add adzuki or black soy beans to our brown rice. About once a week we eat natto. Several times a week we will include some roasted seeds with part of our meal. We will eat either cooked or raw fruit several times a week. We have a small amount of one kind of seaweed most days. For seasonings we use sea salt, shoyu, barley miso, umeboshi, and various vinegars. We drink most herb teas but enjoy bancha or green and brown rice teas most.

In the course of a week, we will use all the various cooking styles: boiling, steaming, pickling, pressing, pressure-cooking, slow stewing, sautéing, grilling, and baking. When the opportunity allows we also have barbecued foods.

Occasional additions

Around this core diet other foods will come and go, depending on what we feel we need at the time, and what is practical and suits us as a family. These include processed grains like pasta, noodles, couscous, bread, polenta, muesli, mochi, or bulgur. We eat most kinds of fish (apart from non-organic farmed fish). Processed foods such as tahini, hummus, nut butters, sugar-free jams, ready made falafels, bean burgers, tofu, tempeh, seiten, pesto sauce, organic healthy biscuits, roasted nuts, olives. We occasionally have fermented dairy

listen to your body

Macrobiotic foods will, over time, change your internal energy, which will lead to your body becoming more attuned to what it needs. It's important that you listen to your body's needs and adapt your diet.

foods such as yogurt, soft cheese, or butter. Once a month or so we might include an egg in a dish. Sometimes we add mustard, black pepper, wasabi, shichimi, shiso powder, tekka, or rice wine to a dish. We might drink juices, hot water with lemon, have the occasional coffee for mental stimulation, use rice, oat, or nut milks, enjoy some wine or beer.

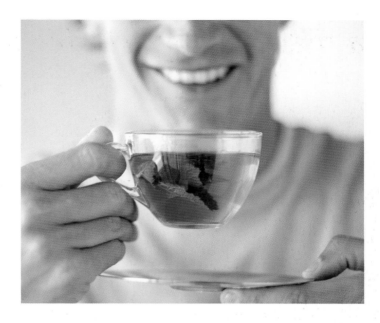

It is important to know which oils are best to use in cooking (see pages 68–71) as many break down at high temperatures, risking oxidization and introducing free radicals into the blood. We use sesame or olive oil for sautéing. Adding oils to soups or stews is safer as they can only reach 225°F. When using raw oils for salad dressings and the like, we have a much wider choice.

I decided not to eat meat 25 years ago, primarily because I did not want to take in the energy of an animal that had recently been slaughtered. Despite my urging them to try it, none of my family eats meat. If they were keen to do so, I would recommend meat such as pheasant, duck, rabbit, or organic meat from a reputable source.

We do not eat any irradiated foods, genetically modified foods or foods that contain additives, colorings, or excessive sugar.

6 steps to macrobiotics

1 Decide whether you are prepared to make organic foods a priority.

2 Make a list of the core ingredients you want to include on a regular basis.

3 Write out all the cooking styles you want to experience weekly.

4 Consider the foods you might have from time to time for convenience, taste, or practicality.

5 Decide which oils to use for cooking.

6 List any foods you want to avoid completely.

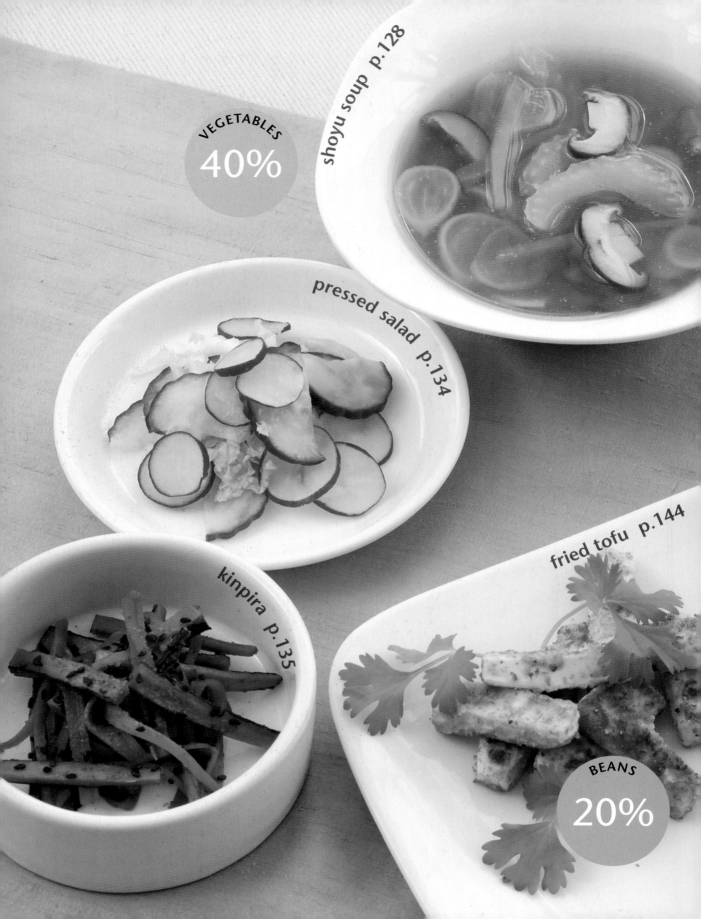

VEGETABLES

40%

shoyu soup p.128

pressed salad p.134

kinpira p.135

fried tofu p.144

BEANS

20%

macrobiotic
recipes for life

The following recipes are all ones I enjoy and use regularly. Remember, macrobiotics is not a prescriptive diet; to get the most benefit from it, you must vary your eating habits and listen to your body – very soon you will intuitively know what it needs for good health.

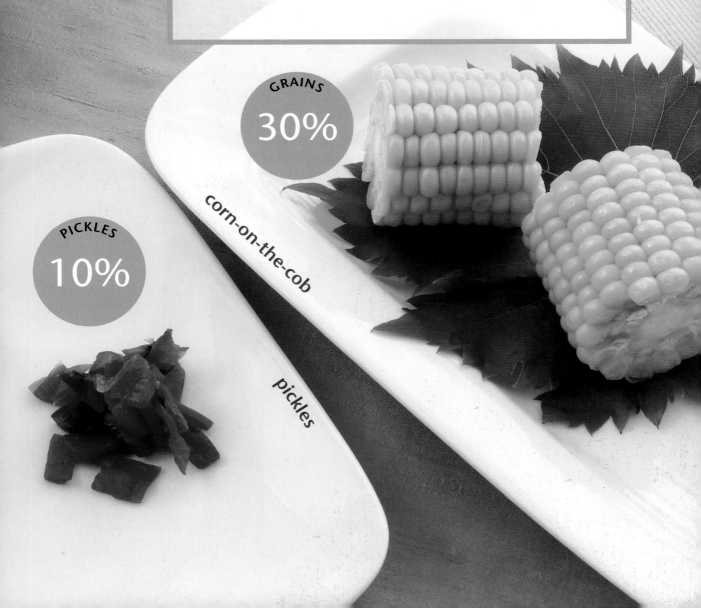

GRAINS
30%

corn-on-the-cob

PICKLES
10%

pickles

breakfast

miso soup

Light and easily digested at the start of the day. It keeps blood sugar levels balanced.

 Cooks in 10 minutes

1 3-inch wakame seaweed strip
1 tbsp miso paste (barley miso is best)
1 handful of watercress, finely chopped
2 Chinese cabbage leaves, finely chopped
2 sheets nori seaweed, cut into fine strips
½ tsp grated ginger

Pre-soak the wakame strip in a bowl for 2 minutes. Bring 4 cups of water to a boil in a pan and reduce the flame to simmer. Add the wakame strip and simmer for 3 minutes. Put the miso paste in a cup and dilute it with 2 tablespoons of cold water. Add the miso mixture to the pan, stir, and simmer gently for 1 minute.

Add the watercress and Chinese cabbage leaves and turn off the heat. Serve with strips of nori. Add a pinch of grated ginger. Keeps for 1 day.

soft brown rice

Very good if you have had any digestive problems and feel tension in your stomach.

 Cooks in 1 hour

1 cup cooked rice (can be mixed with barley, millet, oats, or rye)
2 cups cold water
1 umeboshi plum

Place all the ingredients in a 2-quart pan and bring to a boil with the lid on. Reduce the flame and simmer, semi-covered, for 30–40 minutes on a low flame. Turn off and leave to stand for another 5–10 minutes.

This dish is best eaten as it is. Although it takes about an hour to cook, this dish doesn't require any attention, which leaves you free to get ready for the day. After 30 minutes' cooking time, check that there is some water left in the pan and add more if necessary. Keeps for 3 days.

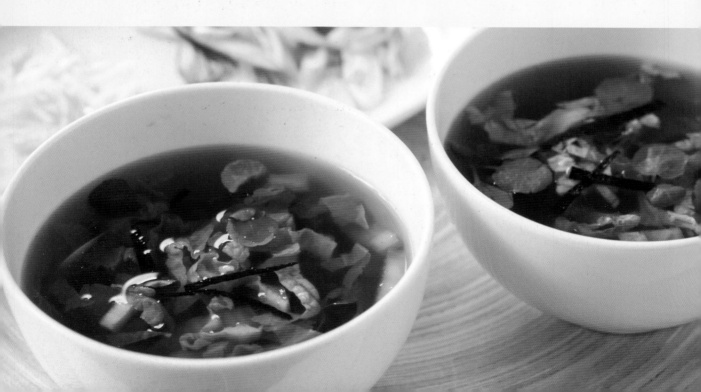

whole oat cereal with kombu, seeds, and nuts

Helps you feel warm and gives lasting energy.

 Cooks in 2 hours 10 minutes

1 cup whole oats soaked overnight in 5 cups water
One 2-inch strip kombu, soaked with the oats
4 tbsp toasted sunflower seeds
4 tbsp toasted chopped almonds

Bring the oats and kombu to a boil in a 3 quart covered pan. Reduce the flame and simmer, uncovered, for 2 hours. Switch off the heat and leave to stand overnight.

In the morning, heat the porridge carefully, making sure there's water in the pan to prevent it from sticking. Add more water if necessary. Serve with 1 tbsp toasted sesame seeds and 1 tbsp toasted almonds in each bowl. Keeps for 3 days.

Steel cut oats with nori

Leaves a long-lasting warm, settled feeling in the abdomen.

  Cooks in 25 minutes

1 cup steel cut oats
¼ cup raisins, rinsed
2 sheets toasted nori, cut into 1-inch strips
2 tbsp toasted sesame seeds

Wash the oats and soak them overnight in 4 cups cold water. In the morning, bring the oats and the water to a boil in a 3-quart covered pan. Reduce the heat and simmer, uncovered, for 15 minutes.

Add the raisins and cook for another 5 minutes, stirring occasionally to stop the ingredients from sticking. Turn off the heat and serve with the strips of nori, sprinkled with the sesame seeds. Keeps for 2 days

fried mochi savory

A warming compact breakfast that contains surprisingly long-lasting energy.

 Cooks in 8 minutes

2 tbsp sesame or olive oil for frying
1 block mochi cut into 12 pieces

FOR THE DRESSING:
1 tbsp natural sauerkraut
1 tbsp fine freshly grated daikon
10 drops (1 tsp) shoyu
1 tsp brown rice vinegar
1 tbsp cold water
½ tsp nori flakes

Warm a cast-iron frying pan with a lid over a low flame for about 1 minute. Add the oil, bring the flame to medium and heat for about 30 seconds. Add the mochi and fry on each side for 2–3 minutes with the lid on, until the mochi puffs up.

Place a few pieces of mochi on each plate. Mix together the dressing ingredients and serve ½ tsp on each mochi. Eat immediately

fried mochi with syrup

A light, satisfying breakfast that lifts your energy.

  Cooks in 8 minutes

2 tbsp sesame or olive oil for frying
1 block mochi, cut into 12 pieces

FOR THE SWEET SAUCE:
2 tbsp rice syrup
1 tbsp maple syrup
few drops of freshly squeezed lemon juice

Prepare the mochi as in the recipe above. Heat the rice and maple syrups in a small pan until it starts to bubble. Serve ½ tsp on each mochi and top with 3–5 drops lemon juice. Eat immediately.

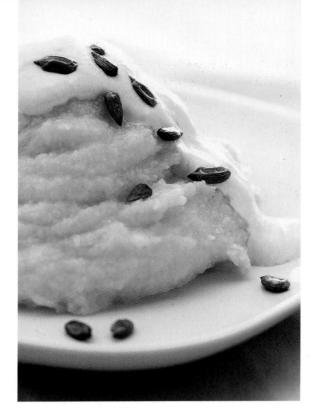

creamy polenta with sunflower seeds and yogurt

A light, refreshing, uplifting breakfast.

  Cooks in 20 minutes

½ **cup organic polenta**
½ **cup yogurt**
¼ **cup sunflower seeds**
sesame oil

Place the polenta and 4 cups cold water in a large pan. Cover, and bring to a boil. When the water is boiling, reduce the heat and put a flame diffuser under the pan. Uncover the pan and simmer for 10–15 minutes, stirring occasionally. Switch off the heat and divide the polenta between 4 serving bowls.

Meanwhile, heat a few drops of sesame oil in a heavy-based frying pan. Add the sunflower seeds and roast, stirring occasionally, until the seeds are brown. Top each bowl with yogurt and a sprinkling of sunflower seeds. Keeps for 1 day.

couscous with sunflower seeds and syrup

A rich, tasty breakfast that helps you feel relaxed.

  Cooks in 20 minutes

¾ **cup couscous**
¼ **cup oatmeal**
1 **tbsp tahini**
1 **medium orange, freshly squeezed**
½ **tsp sesame or sunflower oil**
dry-roasted sunflower seeds, to decorate

Put the couscous and oats in a large pan with 3 cups cold water. Cover and leave to stand overnight.

In the morning, bring the couscous and water to a boil, then simmer for 5 minutes on a low-medium heat. Add the tahini and cook for another 2–3 minutes. Turn off the heat and mix in the orange juice and oil. Sprinkle the sunflower seeds over the couscous and serve. Keeps for 1 day.

polenta with syrup

Light and sweet breakfast for when you want to relax.

  Cooks in 30 minutes

1 **cup organic polenta**
4 **tbsp toasted sesame seeds**
maple syrup (to taste)

Put the polenta and 4 cups cold water into a pan. Bring to a boil, then simmer, uncovered, for 10–15 minutes. Add the seeds and stir. Divide between 4 bowls and add syrup to taste. Keeps for 2 days.

scrambled tofu

A good dish for boosting your energy without upsetting your blood sugar balance.

 Cooks in 12 minutes

1 tbsp sesame oil
1 small onion, coarsely grated
1 small carrot, coarsely grated
½ cup button mushrooms, finely sliced
1 block organic tofu
1½ tbsp shoyu (or to taste)
½ tsp turmeric
2 small scallions, finely chopped

Heat the oil in a medium-sized, heavy-based frying pan over a medium to high heat. Add the onion and carrot and stir for 1–2 minutes. Add the mushrooms and sauté for a further 2 minutes.

Crumble the tofu and add to the frying pan. Cook for 3–4 minutes until all the flavors mix in. Season with shoyu and turmeric, and cook for another minute.

Turn off the heat and place the mixture in a serving dish sprinkled with the chopped scallions. Serve with steamed sourdough bread spread with a thin layer of mustard. Eat immediately.

steamed sourdough bread with hummus and sauerkraut

Good, slow-burning fuel for the morning.

 Cooks in 5 minutes

8 slices of sourdough bread
1 container hummus
8 tbsp natural sauerkraut

Put ½ cup water in a pan. Cover, and bring to a boil. Remove the lid and put a bamboo steamer on top. Place the bread in the steamer and cover.

Steam for 3–4 minutes over a low heat. Remove the bread and put it on a serving plate. Spread each slice with a generous layer of hummus and top with 1 tbsp sauerkraut. Eat immediately.

tahini and jam

Slows your energy, helping you feel secure and stable.

  Cooks in 5 minutes

8 slices of sourdough bread
8 tsp light tahini
8 tsp sugar-free jam

Place ½ cup water in a pan and bring to a boil. Position a bamboo steamer on top. Place the bread in the steamer, cover and steam for 3–4 minutes over a low heat.

Remove the bread and put it on a serving plate. Spread with tahini and top with a layer of your favorite jam. Eat immediately.

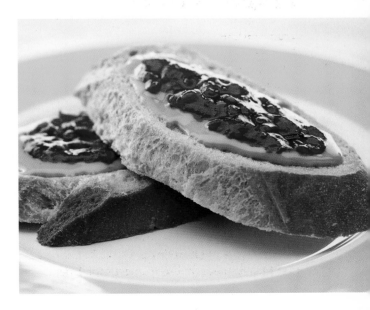

soups

vegetable soup with miso

Increases the flow of energy up and down your body helping you feel upright and independent.

 Cooks in 10 minutes

1 3-inch wakame seaweed strip
1 carrot, washed and finely sliced
1 leek, washed and finely sliced
1 tbsp miso paste (barley miso is best)
2 sheets of nori seaweed, cut into fine strips
½ tsp grated ginger
2 cups clams (optional)

Pre-soak the wakame strip in a bowl for 2 minutes. In a large pan, bring 4 cups water to a boil and reduce the flame to simmer.

Add the carrots and leeks and simmer for 5 minutes. Add the wakame strip and its soaking water. Put the miso paste in a cup and dilute it with 2 tbsp cold water. Add in the miso mixture to the pan and simmer gently for 1 minute.

Serve with strips of nori and a pinch of grated ginger. If you include seafood in the recipe, add the clams with the carrots and leeks. Keeps for 1 day.

barley soup

Barley is the best whole grain for feeling lighter, cleaner, and increasing long-term energy.

  Cooks in 30 minutes

½ cup barley, washed
1 carrot, cut into small squares
1 stalk celery, cut into small squares
½ garlic clove, crushed
1 tbsp olive or sesame oil
sea salt to taste
parsley for seasoning

Place the barley and 2 cups water in a large heavy-based pan and simmer for 10–15 minutes. Turn off the heat and allow to soak overnight.

Put the vegetables, barley, and twice as much water in a pan and bring to a boil. Simmer for 15–20 minutes. Add the garlic, oil, and sea salt. Simmer for another 5 minutes, decorate with parsley leaves and serve. Keeps for 2–3 days.

lentil soup

A well-balanced soup that's a meal in itself.

  Cooks in 20 minutes

1 cup green lentils
2 celery stalks, diced
1 medium carrot, diced
2 bay leaves
1 tsp sea salt
2 tbsp sunflower oil
½ tsp turmeric
½ tsp cumin
5 fresh shiitake mushrooms, sliced
3 small scallions, finely diced
4 lemon slices (to garnish)

Wash the lentils, then soak them overnight in 2 cups warm water. The following day, bring them to a boil in the same water and cook for 10 minutes.

Meanwhile, place the celery, carrot, and lentils in a cast-iron pan. Add the bay leaves and 4–6 cups water. Cover. Bring to a boil. Reduce the flame to medium and cook for 15–20 minutes. Halfway through, add the salt.

Heat the oil in a pan. Add the mushrooms and scallions and sauté for 1 minute. Add the turmeric and cumin and sauté for a further 1–2 minutes. Pour the mixture into the soup and simmer for 2 minutes. Serve with a slice of lemon. Keeps for 2 days.

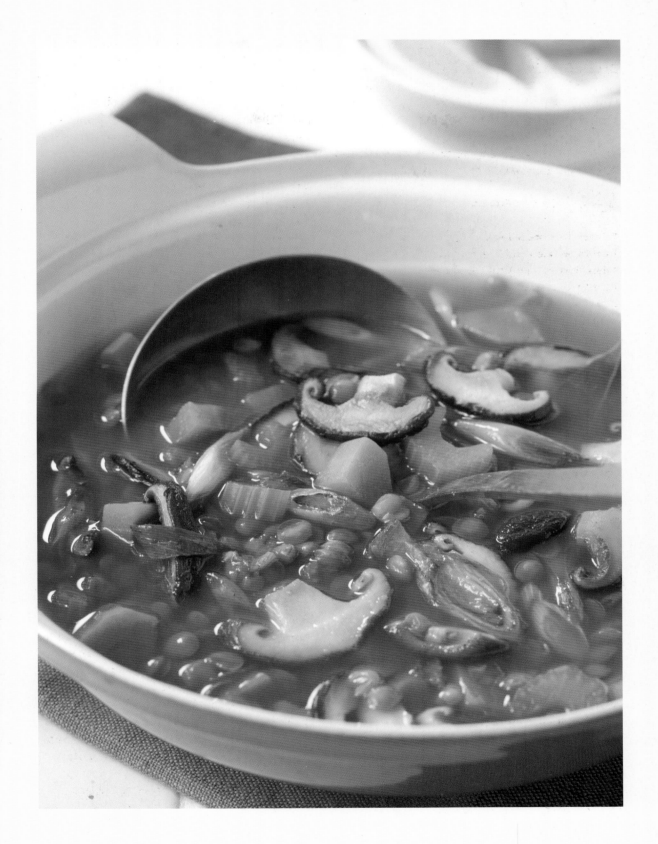

shoyu soup with carrot and radish

Helps you feel lighter and cleaner inside.

 Cooks in 18 minutes

1-inch piece dried kombu
4 dried shiitake mushrooms
1 carrot, cut into fine strips
1 stalk celery, cut in thin, diagonal strips
1 bunch radishes, thinly sliced
1 tbsp shoyu (to taste)
nori, cut into strips, for decoration

Pour 4 cups cold water into a large pan and bring to a boil. Add the kombu and mushrooms and simmer for about 10 minutes.

Remove the kombu and mushrooms from the pan, and slice the mushrooms thinly, discarding the stalks. Put them back in the pan together with the carrot, celery, and radishes. Season with shoyu to taste and simmer for another minute.

Turn off the heat and leave the soup to stand for 3–4 minutes. This allows the vegetables to cook for a little longer, but they will still have some bite. Garnish with the nori just before serving. Keeps for 2 days.

sweet millet soup

Leaves a warm, nourished feeling in your abdomen.

  Cooks in 35 minutes

½ cup millet, washed
½ cup ripe sweet squash (Japanese kabocha is best), cut into chunks
1 carrot, cut into small chunks
1 small parsnip, cut into small chunks
1 small onion, cut into small chunks
½-1 tsp sea salt
1 scallion, finely sliced diagonally (to garnish)

Dry-roast the millet in a large frying pan until it turns a golden color.

Place the squash, carrot, parsnips, and onion on top of the millet. Cover with water and season with salt. Bring to a boil, lower the flame, and simmer for 20–30 minutes, checking occasionally to make sure that the millet, which absorbs a lot of water, is always covered with water.

When the millet is soft, switch off the heat. Garnish with scallion and serve. Keeps for 2 days.

clear cauliflower soup

A clean-tasting soup that makes you feel lighter.

 Cooks in 15 minutes

1-inch piece dried wakame
1 cauliflower, cut into florets
½ tsp shoyu (or to taste)
1 sheet nori, cut into 1-inch fine strips
parsley, for decoration

Place the wakame in a bowl and soak in ¼ cup water for 5 minutes. Remove the wakame, reserving the soaking water, and chop into small pieces. Pour the reserved water into a measuring jug and top up to 4 cups with cold water. Pour the liquid into a large pan and add the cauliflower florets.

Cover the pan and bring to a boil, then reduce the heat to medium and simmer for 5 minutes. Add the wakame and simmer for a further 2–3 minutes. Season with shoyu and add the nori. Simmer for 1 more minute, then turn off the heat. Serve garnished with parsley. Keeps for 1 day.

cucumber and ginger soup

A light, refreshing soup that helps you feel clean inside.

  Cooks in 20 minutes

5 dried shiitake mushrooms
1-inch piece kombu
1 tbsp olive or sesame oil
1 bunch scallions, cut diagonally into thin pieces
1-inch piece ginger, cut into matchsticks
sea salt
1 cucumber, washed, peeled, halved, and cut into thin half-moon slices
½ block tofu, cut into small squares
2 tbsp cornstarch
fresh cilantro, for decoration

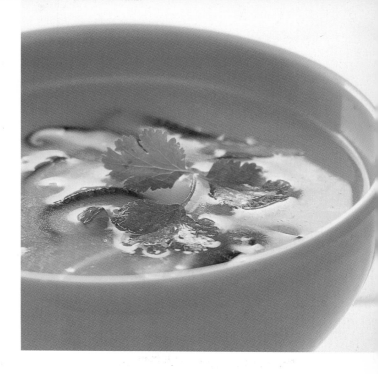

Pre-soak the shiitake mushrooms and kombu in ½ cup cold water for 5–10 minutes. Reserve the soaking water. Discard the stems from the mushrooms. Cut the mushrooms and the kombu into squares.

Heat the oil in a large pan. Add the scallions and ginger and stir with a pair of chopsticks. Dip the chopsticks into sea salt and use them to stir the onions and ginger over a high heat for about a minute. Add the mushrooms and cucumber and sauté for another minute. Now add the kombu, the reserved soaking water, and the tofu, and simmer for about 2–3 minutes. Pour in 3–4 cups water, cover, and bring to a boil. Meanwhile, mix the cornstarch with ¼ cup cold water to make a paste.

As soon as the soup boils, remove the lid, add the corn starch mixture and 1 tsp sea salt and simmer over a very low heat for a few minutes. Garnish with fresh cilantro. Keeps for 1 day.

pea, celery, and mint soup

A light, refreshing soup that helps you feel "up."

  Cooks in 25 minutes

1 tbsp olive oil
1 large or 2 small onions, chopped
sea salt
½ kg green peas
1–2 stalks celery, roughly chopped
handful of mint, finely chopped

Heat the oil in a large pan, add the chopped onion and sauté for 1 minute, stirring with a pair of chopsticks. Dip the chopsticks in the sea salt and stir the onion again. Add the peas and celery and 4 tbsp water. Cover the pan and continue cooking for 1 minute.

Add 3–4 cups water to the pan, bring to a boil, then reduce the heat to medium and simmer for 15 minutes. Stir in the mint. Turn off the heat, liquidize the soup in a food processor, then return it to the pan. Leave to stand for 5 minutes before serving. Keeps for 2 days.

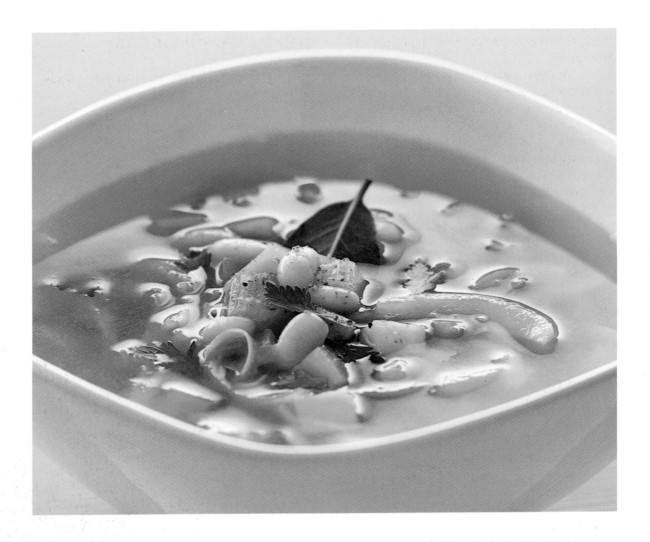

bean and vegetable soup

A warming soup that spreads warmth and strength from your abdomen.

  Cooks in 55 minutes

1 cup dried haricot beans (or organic sugar-free
 tinned beans)
3 bay leaves
1 small onion, sliced
1 carrot, diced
1 stalk celery, diced
1 parsnip, diced
1 tsp sea salt
2 tbsp olive oil
1 tbsp organic unbleached white flour,
 (wheat or rice)
1 tsp shichimi (also known as seven-spice)
flat-leaf parsley, for decoration

If you are using dried beans, prepare them a day in advance by rinsing and then placing them in a large, covered pan with 3 cups warm water. Soak the beans overnight.

 When ready to use, heat the beans and water and bring to a boil. Boil for a couple of minutes, then drain and discard the water. Rinse the beans and place in a large saucepan. Add 4 cups water, the bay leaves and onion and bring to a boil.

Cook, covered, over a high heat for about 10 minutes.

Add the carrot, celery, and parsnip to the beans. Lower the heat to medium and simmer for another 30 minutes, with the lid slightly to one side so that the steam can escape easily. About halfway through the cooking time, add a further cup of water and the sea salt.

Meanwhile, put the oil and flour in a small pan, heat gently and stir constantly for about 2 minutes so the flour does not burn. Add the mixture to the beans, stir well and simmer for another 2 minutes. Before serving, put a pinch of shichimi in each soup bowl and then add the soup. Decorate with the flat-leaf parsley. Keeps for 2 days.

carrot soup

A grounding soup for when you need to be practical.

 Cooks in 25 minutes

1 tbsp olive or sesame oil
1 medium onion, cut into squares
4 carrots, washed and cut into large chunks
½ cauliflower
½ tsp sea salt
¼ tsp cumin
4 cups water
1 cup leftover cooked oats (or rice)

Heat the oil in a pan, add the onion and sauté for 2 minutes. Add the carrots, cauliflower, sea salt, and cumin. Add the water slowly and bring to a boil, covered. Reduce the flame to medium-low and cook for about 15 minutes.

Liquidize the soup in a blender, then return it to the pan, adding more water if it is too thick. Add the leftover oats or rice. Simmer for 1 minute and serve. Keeps for 1–2 days.

potato and carrot soup

A warming and comforting soup that aids feelings of contentment.

  Cooks in 20 minutes

8 medium potatoes, peeled and cut into small squares
2 carrots cut into slightly bigger squares than the potatoes
1 tbsp olive oil
1 tsp sea salt (or to taste)
¼ tsp white pepper
2 cups Chinese cabbage, cut into slices

Put the potatoes and about 6 cups water into a pan. Bring to a boil and simmer for 5–10 minutes. Add the carrots and cook for a further 5–10 minutes. Add oil, sea salt, and pepper. Simmer for a minute, switch off and add the Chinese cabbage. Serve with some flat-leaf parsley. Keeps for 1 day.

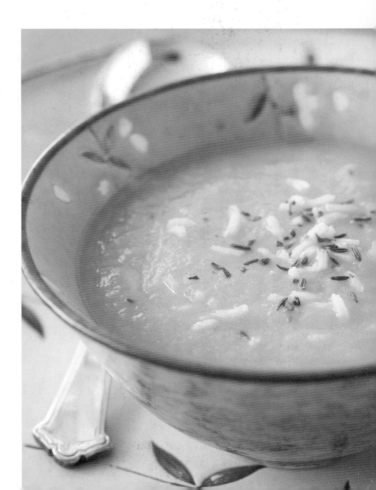

main meals

brown rice and whole grains

Whole grains are staple foods in macrobiotics, providing a good range of nutrition that is easy to digest.

 Cooks in 1 hour, plus soaking

¼ **cup barley, wheat, rye, oats, or spelt**
1½ **cups short-grain brown rice**
¼ **cup whole adzuki, soy, or kidney beans**
½ **tsp sea salt or strip of kombu**

Put the grains and beans into a pressure-cooker. Wash and rinse a few times with cold water. Add 2¾ cups spring water and leave the mixture to soak overnight.

The next day, add the salt or kombu, put the lid on tight and bring to a boil slowly, over a medium flame, to avoid burning. Place the flame diffuser on another ring, warm it up and, when the pressure valve pops up, put the rice on the diffuser. Pressure-cook it for 40 minutes from the moment the pressure valve comes up. When finished, switch off, remove from the diffuser and, as soon as the pressure valve comes down, remove the lid and transfer the rice in a pre-rinsed bowl. Leave to cool. Keeps for 3 days.

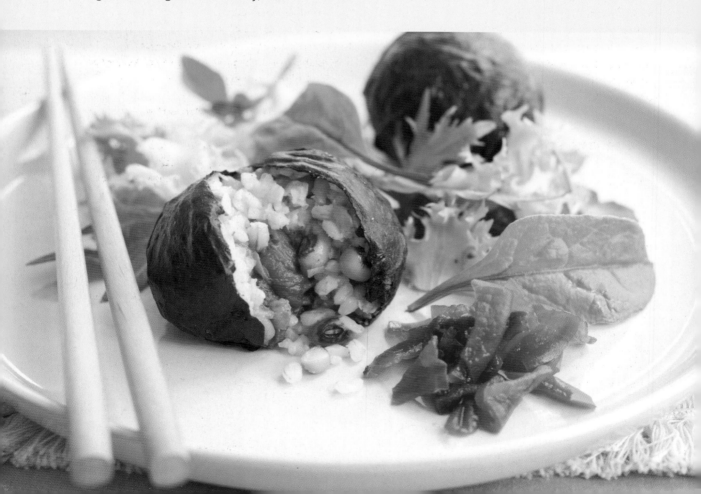

Japanese rice balls

Combines the goodness of the whole grains with the flavor of the sea vegetable.

 Prepare in 10 minutes

4 sheets nori sea vegetable, pre-toasted if possible
2 cups brown rice and whole grains (see page 132)
2 umeboshi plums

Take the sheets of nori and, if they are not pre-toasted, drag them over a flame quickly until they become lighter green in color. Cut into quarters and lay out on a dry board.

Wet your hands and pick up a handful of the rice and whole grain mixture to form a ball (wet your hands each time you do this to prevent the rice from sticking.) Press about a quarter of an umeboshi plum into the whole grain mixture and seal the hole with more whole grains.

Lay the ball onto one sheet of nori and place another sheet on top. Shape so that the corners are between the corners of the lower sheet. Press the corners onto the sides of the ball. Finally, pick up the rice ball and squeeze so that all the nori sticks to the rice. Serve 2 rice balls per person on a bed of salad. Keeps for 1 day.

millet mash

A warm, satisfying dish that relaxes your abdomen.

  Cooks in 30 minutes

½ cup millet, washed
1 small onion
1 small carrot, cut into little chunks
½ parsnip, cut into little chunks
½ cup sweet squash (Japanese kabocha is best), cut into chunks
½–1 tsp sea salt
1 small scallion, very finely sliced diagonally, for decoration

Dry-roast the millet in a heavy frying pan until it turns golden.

In a large, heavy-based pan, layer the onions, carrots, parsnip, and pumpkin, with the millet on top. Cover with water, season with sea salt, and bring to a boil on a low to medium flame. Simmer on a low flame for about 20 minutes, checking occasionally to make sure that the millet, which absorbs a great deal of water, is always covered with water.

Once the millet is cooked (it should be soft), switch off and serve garnished with scallions. Keeps for 1 day.

garlic rice

Takes the strenghening qualities of brown rice and adds a strong, fiery, expansive component.

  Cooks in 7 minutes

1–2 tsp olive or sesame oil
1 tsp ginger, very finely chopped
2–3 cloves of garlic, very finely chopped
2 cups short-grain organic rice (pre-cooked, either boiled or pressure cooked)
sea salt
parsley, finely chopped, for decoration

Heat the oil in a stainless steel wok or large frying pan. Add the ginger and garlic, stirring constantly. Then add the cooked rice and stir quickly over a high heat with a long wooden spatula for a few minutes. You may have to add very small amounts of water occasionally to stop the ingredients from burning. Add the salt and stir for another couple of minutes.

Switch off the heat, mix thoroughly and transfer into a serving dish. Garnish with parsley and serve. Eat immediately.

pressed cucumber, Chinese cabbage, and radish salad

A clean, sharp-tasting, refreshing dish.

  Cooks in 20 minutes

1 small cucumber, cut in half then thinly sliced
2 cups Chinese cabbage, finely sliced
3–4 radishes, thinly sliced diagonally
¼ tsp sea salt

Place the cucumber, cabbage, and radishes in a deep bowl, sprinkle over the salt, and mix gently with your hands for a minute. Put a flat plate on top of the ingredients within the bowl, and weigh it down with a jug of water. Leave to stand for 10–15 minutes.

Remove the jug and, holding the plate firmly in place, drain the liquid from the vegetables over the sink. Place the pressed ingredients in a serving bowl and serve. Eat immediately.

Chinese cabbage and sauerkraut rolls

A refreshing, crunchy dish with good cleansing properties.

  Cooks in 10 minutes

4 large Chinese cabbage leaves
4 tbsp ready made sauerkraut

In a large steamer, bring a little cold water to a boil. Place the cabbage leaves in the steamer and steam for approximately 4 minutes. Allow the leaves to cool.

Place the leaves on a flat surface with the inner part facing upward. In the middle of each leaf, put 1 tbsp sauerkraut, then roll up the leaf, starting from the stem end. Squeeze each leaf gently to get rid of any excess liquid. Eat immediately.

adzuki bean and root vegetable stew

A strengthening and relaxing stew.

  Cooks in 1 hour

1-inch strip kombu
2–3 cups Hokkaido pumpkin or carrots or parsnips (or a combination), washed and cut into chunks
1 cup adzuki beans, soaked for at least 3 hours
1–2 tsp shoyu
1 scallion, chopped, to garnish

Layer the kombu, vegetables, and beans in a pan. Add enough water to cover the contents. Simmer, covered, for 40 minutes or until the beans are soft, adding water occasionally to keep the contents covered. Turn off the heat and add shoyu to taste. Garnish with scallions. Keeps for 2 days.

nishime

A grounding dish, ideal for greater perserverance.

  Cooks in 35 minutes

1-inch piece kombu
1 medium onion, peeled and cut into quarters
½ cup pumpkin, scrubbed but unpeeled, cut into big chunks (optional)
1 carrot, scrubbed and cut into chunks
1 parsnip, scrubbed and cut into chunks
pinch sea salt
1 tsp shoyu

Place the kombu into a large, heavy-based pan and then layer the vegetables on top. Add ½ cup cold water, taking care not to "disturb" the vegetables. Sprinkle over a pinch of sea salt, cover, and bring to a boil. Reduce the heat to medium and cook for 20–30 minutes. There should be a little water covering the base of the pan. Season with shoyu, replace the lid, and simmer for another minute before serving. Keeps for 1 day.

blanched vegetables

A refreshing dish that encourages your energy to rise.

  Cooks in 6 minutes

1 cup cabbage, cut into small squares
1 carrot, cut diagonally into thin pieces
1 cup broccoli, cut into small florets
1 cup cauliflower, cut into small florets
1 cup kale, cut into thin slices
ume vinegar, to taste

Put 2–3 cups water in a large pan and bring to a boil. Add the cabbage and blanch for 1 minute. Remove using a slotted spoon and place on a plate. Repeat with the carrots, broccoli, cauliflower, and kale. Allow the vegetables to cool.

Place the vegetables in a serving dish and add ume vinegar to taste. Eat immediately.

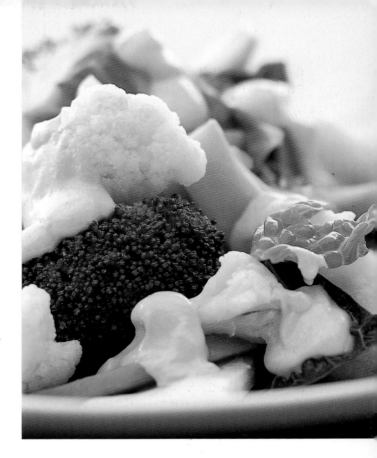

kinpira

Ideal for increasing flexibility and tenacity.

  Cooks in 20 minutes

1 tsp toasted sesame or olive oil
2 pieces burdock (gently scrubbed but unpeeled),
   cut into thin shavings or matchsticks
2 carrots, cut into thin shavings
1 tbsp mirin (optional)
1 tbsp shoyu
¼ tsp shichimi
1 tsp black sesame seeds, dry-pan fried

Heat the oil in a heavy-based pan. Sauté the burdock for 2 minutes. Add the carrots and sauté for 1 minute. Add the mirin and ½ cup cold water. Cover and simmer on a medium to high heat for 5–7 minutes, adding a little water if necessary.

Add the shoyu and simmer for another minute. Switch off the heat and add the shichimi. Leave to stand, covered, for a couple of minutes then serve sprinkled with sesame seeds. Keeps for 1 day.

steamed vegetables

Ideal for stirring up the energy around your liver and lungs.

 Cooks in 5 minutes

Watercress, Chinese cabbage, bok choy, chard,
   radish tops, kale, or cabbage (or a combination),
   cut into thin strips
1 large carrot, cut into thin strips along its length
4 radishes, halved
1 tsp shoyu
1 tsp brown rice vinegar

Place the vegetables in a steamer and steam over boiling water for about 2 minutes. Place on a serving dish and sprinkle with shoyu and vinegar. Eat immediately.

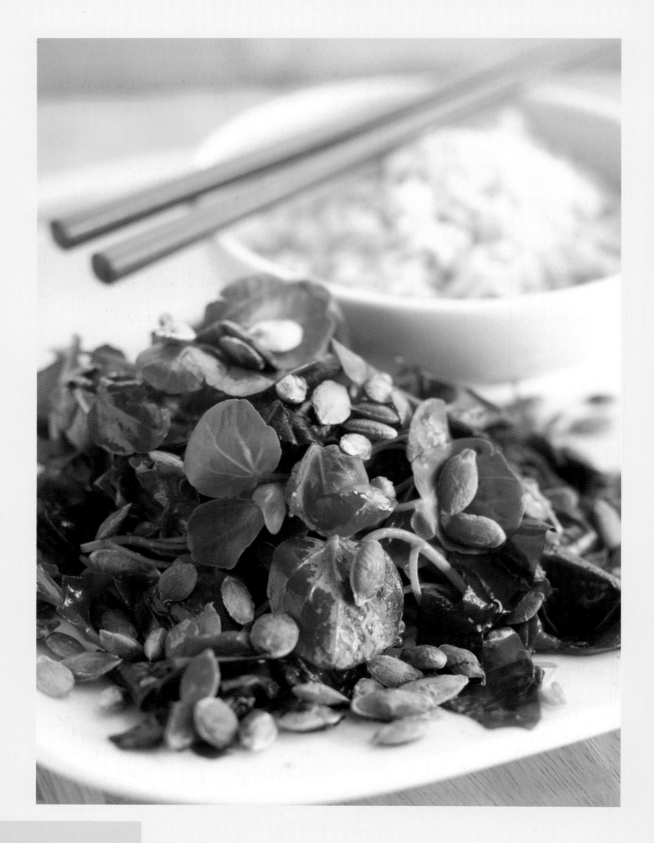

quickly pickled radishes

A sharp taste that refreshes and cleans the body.

 Cooks in 12 minutes

1 bunch radishes, trimmed and finely sliced
2 tbsps umeboshi vinegar

Place the radish slices in a deep, flat bowl. In a small pan, add the vinegar to 1 cup water and bring the mixture to a boil. Remove from the heat and pour over the radishes. Leave to stand for 10 minutes.

When serving, drain the radishes and place them on a serving dish, reserving the vinegar mixture to use later in salad dressings. The radishes will keep in the vinegar mixture for 3 days.

watercress and dulse salad

A mineral-rich dish and a good blood tonic.

 Cooks in 10 minutes

1 6-inch dulse strip
2 tbsp pumpkin seeds, washed
1 tbsp olive oil
1 bunch watercress, washed and roughly chopped
1 tbsp shoyu

Dip the dulse in water and leave it to go soft. Meanwhile, toast the pumpkin seeds in a lightly oiled frying pan over a medium heat, stirring frequently to prevent burning, until light brown. Leave the seeds on a plate to cool.

Cut the dulse into thin slices. Pour just enough water to cover the surface into the frying pan. Heat the water, add the dulse and soften, then drain the water. Add the watercress and sauté for 1–2 minutes, stirring occasionally.

Turn off the heat, season with shoyu, and transfer to a serving bowl. Mix in the pumpkin seeds before serving. Eat immediately.

barley stew

A rich, hearty, strengthening stew that moves your energy up.

  Cooks in 1 hour 40 minutes, plus soaking

1 cup barley, washed and pre-soaked in cold water for 2–3 hours or overnight
2 carrots, diced
1 diced leek
1 stalk celery, diced
sea salt
olive or sesame oil
4 slices sourdough rice or barley bread
1 clove garlic, halved
fresh flat-leaf parsley, for decoration

Place the barley in a large pan and cover with water to twice the barley's depth. Cook for 20–30 minutes, checking occasionally to make sure there is enough water in the pan.

In another heavy-based pan, layer the vegetables and barley in the following order: carrot, leek, celery, barley. Cover with twice as much water and cook on a medium–low heat for 40–60 minutes, adding water occasionally.

Season with sea salt. (Always add a small amount, taste and then add more, if necessary.) Simmer for a further 10 minutes, turn off the heat and cover the pan. The stew should be creamy and moist, not watery.

In a frying pan (preferably cast-iron), pour just enough oil to cover the surface. Fry each slice of bread for a couple of minutes on each side on a medium to high heat. Remove the bread and rub the cut garlic clove on both sides of the bread.

To serve, put the bread slices in a serving bowl and add the stew on top. If you like, decorate with a few parsley leaves. Keeps for 3 days.

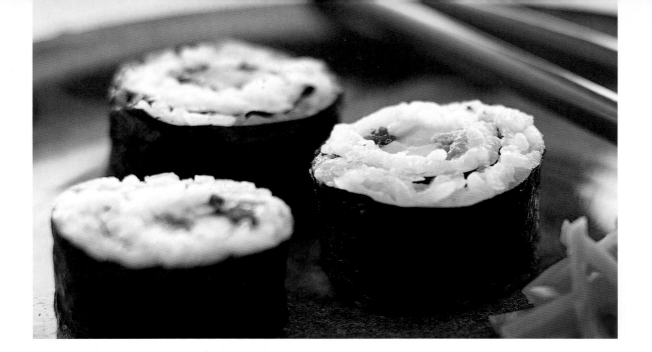

sushi

A meal in itself, great food for when you're on the move.

 Cooks in 15 minutes

1–2 cups sushi rice (leftover rice is ideal)
10 sheets of nori
1 tbsp tahini (sesame seed paste)
1 tbsp umeboshi paste
1–2 tbsp sauerkraut
1 carrot, cut into long matchsticks
1 tsp wasabi powder
shoyu, to taste
pickled ginger slices, to serve

Cook the rice according to the packet instructions, then leave to one side to cool down.

Lay a sheet of nori, rough side up, on a sushi mat or flat surface. Dip a spatula into a jug of water and use the wet spatula to spread some rice over the nori (do this each time you add more rice to stop the rice from sticking to the spatula).

Spread the rice with a little tahini, a tiny amount of umeboshi paste and a little sauerkraut. Lay a few carrot matchsticks down the center and, using the mat as a guide, roll up the sushi as if making a Swiss roll.

Use a wet knife to cut it into eight slices. Repeat as above with the remaining ingredients.

To make wasabi paste in which to dip the sushi, put the wasabi powder in a small dish and add a little water at a time. If you add too much water, you will need to add more wasabi. When you have a thick paste, divide it between the serving plates.

Spoon a little shoyu onto each plate. Serve the sushi with a few slices of pickled ginger. Keeps for 1 day.

emerald eye stew

A light summer dish that helps you feel energized.

  Cooks in 15 minutes

3 dried shiitake mushrooms
2 tbsp white miso
2 tbsp shoyu
1-inch piece ginger, unpeeled and cut into
  4–5 thin slices
15 runner or green beans
1 head broccoli, cut into florets

1 tbsp olive or sesame oil
1 block tofu, cut into small squares
1 small clove garlic, crushed
1 cup bok choy, finely sliced
1 cup watercress, finely chopped
1 Chinese cabbage leaf, finely sliced
1 tbsp arrowroot
cooked couscous, to serve

Place 4 cups water, the mushrooms, miso, shoyu, and ginger slices in a flame-proof casserole. Slowly bring to the boil, then reduce the heat and remove the mushrooms. Cut the stems off and discard, slice the caps and return them to the casserole. Add the beans and broccoli and simmer for 2 minutes.

Meanwhile, heat the oil in a frying pan and fry the tofu for a couple of minutes. Remove the tofu using a slotted spoon and place in the casserole.

Briefly fry the garlic in the frying pan and add it to the stew, along with any remaining oil. Add the bok choy, watercress, and Chinese cabbage to the casserole and turn the heat to low.

In a cup, mix the arrowroot with 2 tbsp cold water and stir until smooth. Add it to the stew, stirring constantly to prevent lumps. It should only take a few minutes for the stew to thicken. Serve on top of cooked couscous. Eat immediately.

natto

A settling and strengthening dish.

 Prepare in 5 minutes

1 container natto
6 tbsp grated daikon, jinengo, or carrot
2 tsp mustard
1 tbsp shoyu

Place all the ingredients in a bowl, mix together thoroughly and serve. Eat immediately.

couscous with tofu and vegetable salad

Brings a light, fresh energy with plenty of variety.

 Cooks in 12 minutes

FOR THE MARINADE:
2 tbsp shoyu
1 tbsp brown rice vinegar

1 block tofu, diced
sea salt
1½ cups couscous
2 tbsp olive or sesame oil
1 onion, diced
1 carrot, diced
1 stalk celery, diced
½ cup peas (fresh or frozen)
½ cup sweet corn kernels (fresh or frozen)
3 tbsp shoyu
chives, for decoration

First make a marinade by mixing the shoyu and vinegar together. Place the squares of tofu into a bowl, cover with the shoyu and vinegar marinade and leave it to stand for about 10 minutes, turning it over occasionally.

Add 2 cups water to a large pan and bring to a boil. Add a pinch of sea salt. Turn off the heat and add the couscous. Cover and leave to soak for 10 minutes.

Meanwhile, heat the oil in a large, heavy-based pan or wok. Add the marinated tofu and onion, and stir with a pair of chopsticks. Dip the tips of the chopsticks into the sea salt, then continue to stir the onion and tofu with them. Fry for a few minutes, stirring continuously. Add the carrots and celery and stir well. Cook for a few minutes more then add the peas and sweet corn. Cook for another 3–4 minutes, then turn off the heat.

Stir in the couscous. Season with the shoyu and garnish with chopped chives. Keeps for 1 day.

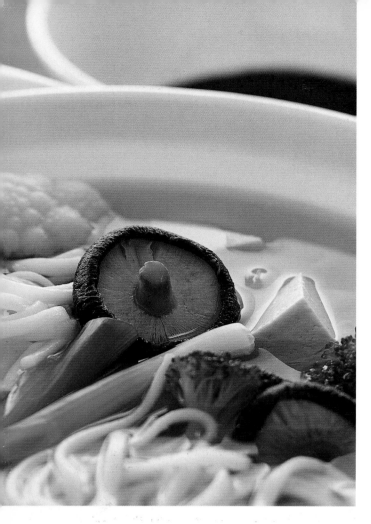

4 small cauliflower florets
½ cup daikon, cut into matchsticks
1 block tofu and/or any white fish

FOR THE SAUCE:
1 tsp black sesame seeds
1 tbsp shoyu
1 tbsp brown rice vinegar
1 tsp ginger, grated

Cook the noodles according to the packet instructions, but leave them slightly underdone (a minute or so less than the recommended cooking time). Drain and reserve.

Meanwhile, prepare the sauce. Wash the sesame seeds under running water. Heat up a frying pan, add the sesame seeds and toast them, stirring constantly until they start to pop (3–5 minutes). Remove from the heat and mix the seeds with the other sauce ingredients.

Fill another large, heavy-based pan or flame-proof casserole with 4–6 cups water. Add the kombu and mushrooms. Bring to a boil, covered, on a medium to high heat. Reduce the heat to very low, remove the kombu and pour the liquid into the nabe dish. Add all the vegetables, tofu, fish, and noodles. Cover the pan and continue cooking on a high flame. When it starts boiling (after about 3–4 minutes), the nabe is ready.

To serve, divide the sauce between 4 serving bowls and add a ladleful of broth from the nabe pot to each. Transfer the nabe pot to the table. Use chopsticks to help yourselves to cooked ingredients from the nabe pot a mouthful at a time, dipping them into the sauce in your bowls as you do so. Eat immediately. This is a complete meal in itself.

nabe

Eating nabe makes you feel hotter, bringing energy from deep inside to the surface quickly.

 Cooks in 30 minutes

1 packet udon (or soba) noodles
1 piece kombu
1–2 dried shiitake mushrooms, pre-soaked and sliced, stems discarded
1 medium carrot, cut diagonally into thin slices
1 small leek, cut diagonally into thin slices
4 scallions, halved
2 Chinese cabbage leaves (or other leafy greens), cut into large squares
4 small broccoli florets

fried rice balls

Contains and strenghtens your energy in a way that greatly increases your stamina.

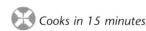 *Cooks in 15 minutes*

4 sheets nori sea vegetable, pre-toasted if possible
4 cups brown rice and whole grains (see page 132)
2 umeboshi plums
8 tsp tahini paste
4 tbsp sesame seeds (brown or black)
olive or sesame oil for frying

FOR THE DIPPING SAUCE:
2 tbsp shoyu
2 tbsp water
1 tbsp brown rice vinegar
1 tsp ginger, finely grated
2 tbsp daikon, finely grated

Take the sheets of nori and, if they are not pre-toasted, drag them over a flame quickly until they become lighter green in color. Cut into quarters and lay out on a dry board.

Wet your hands and mold a handful of the rice and whole grain mixture to form a ball (wet your hands each time you do this to avoid rice sticking). Press about a quarter of an umeboshi plum into the whole grain mixture and seal the hole with more whole grains.

Lay the ball onto one sheet of nori, spread each ball with 1 tsp tahini and sprinkle on sesame seeds. Place another sheet of nori on top and shape so that the corners are between the corners of the lower sheet. Press the corners onto the sides of the ball. Finally, pick up the rice ball and squeeze so that all the nori sticks to the rice.

Add sufficient oil to coat the bottom of a cast-iron frying pan and heat gently. Add the rice balls and fry, turning them gently, until the nori turns slightly brown all over. Place a couple of sheets of kitchen roll on a large plate. Take the rice balls from the pan using a slotted spoon and place on the kitchen paper to remove any excess oil.

Mix all the dipping sauce ingredients together and divide between 4 individual small dishes.

Serve 2 rice balls per person with the dipping sauce. Eat immediately.

soba spice

Although the soba developes inner strength, the frying and spices move your energy outward.

  Cooks in 20 minutes

1 packet soba noodles
1 tbsp sesame oil (or toasted sesame oil in winter)
1 small onion, sliced
1 large carrot, cut into matchsticks
2 stalks celery, sliced
4 Chinese cabbage leaves, sliced
4 tbsp shoyu
2 tbsp grated ginger
1 tsp shichimi, (optional)

Cook the noodles according to the instructions on the packet but cook them *al dente*, so that they are not too soft. Drain and rinse them thoroughly.

Heat the oil in a large wok or frying pan. Add the onion and stir-fry for 1 minute, then add the carrot and celery. Quickly stir-fry for 2 minutes. Add the noodles and mix well with the vegetables. Add the cabbage leaves.

Season with shoyu. Turn off the heat. Squeeze ginger over the mixture and add the shichimi. Eat immediately.

fried polenta

A light, soft dish that feels easy on the stomach.

 Cooks in 15 minutes, plus cooling

sea salt
1 cup polenta (corn grits)
2–3 tbsp cornmeal
sesame oil (for frying)

Place 4 cups cold water and a pinch of sea salt in a large pan. Bring to a boil, then remove from the heat. Slowly whisk the polenta into the water and put the pan back on a low heat, over a flame diffuser. Cover and cook for 10 minutes, whisking once after 5 minutes or so, until thick.

Spoon the polenta onto a baking tray and smooth out using the back of the spoon. Leave to cool (this may take a few hours.)

When nearly ready to serve, cut the polenta into pieces and dip them into the cornmeal. Heat a little oil in a heavy-based frying pan and sauté the pieces for a few minutes on each side, until they are golden brown and crispy. The polenta mixture keeps for 2 days before frying.

seitan dish

A very rich, warming dish that helps you feel content.

  Cooks in 25 minutes

2 tbsp sesame oil
3 medium onions, finely chopped
3 tbsp unbleached white flour
2 medium carrots, cut into small squares
2 cups seitan, finely chopped
1 tsp sea salt
¼ tsp black pepper
2 tbsp parsley, chopped
shichimi (optional)

Heat the oil in a large frying pan. Add the onions and sauté for a couple of minutes. Add the flour and stir for another minute. Add 4 cups water and bring to a boil. Simmer for about 10 minutes. Add the carrots and seitan and cook for another 5–10 minutes. Season with salt and black pepper and add the parsley. Simmer for one minute and turn off the heat.

Serve with potatoes or boiled macaroni. Eat immediately.

noodles

Helps you to feel warm and active.

 Cooks in 20 minutes

1 packet cooked udon or soba noodles
1 2-inch kombu piece
4 small shiitake mushrooms
¼ tsp sea salt
1 cup bonito flakes (optional)
1 small onion, sliced in half-moons
1 small carrot, cut into matchsticks
¼ cup shoyu
1 scallion, finely cut diagonally
2 sheets of nori seaweed, finely cut
shichimi (to taste)

After cooking the noodles according to the packet instructions, drain and rinse them thoroughly and set them aside.

To make the broth, place the kombu, mushrooms, and salt in a large pan with 4 cups water. Bring to a boil on a medium flame. Place the bonito flakes in a sieve over the pan and cover with water. Simmer for 2–3 minutes.

Remove and discard the bonito flakes and kombu. Slice the mushrooms, discarding the stems, and put them back in the pan. Add the onion. Cook for 5 minutes. Add the carrot. Simmer for 2 minutes.

Season with shoyu. Simmer for another couple of minutes and turn off the heat. Serve the noodles and pour over the hot broth. Garnish with scallion and nori. Add the shichimi. Eat immediately.

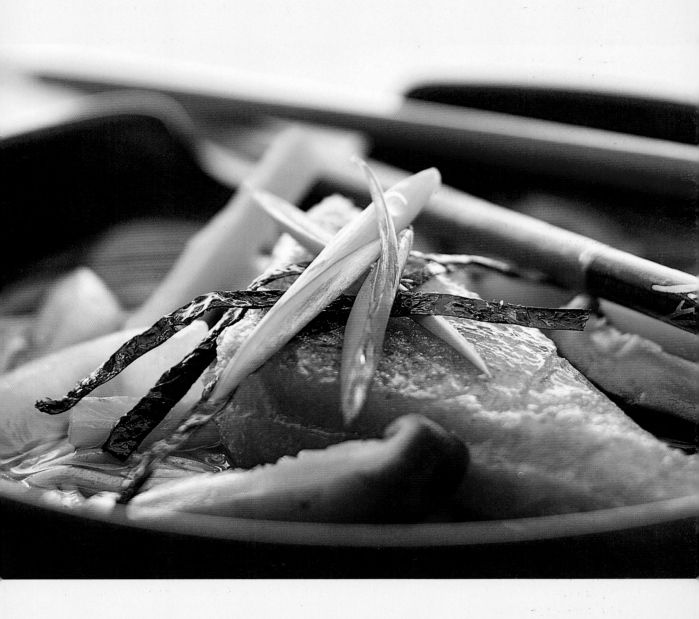

fried tofu or cod

A rich, satisfying dish that is surprisingly light. It helps warm and move your energy outward.

 Cooks in 10 minutes

3–4 tsp olive or sesame oil
6 tsp wholemeal flour
1 block organic tofu, drained and cut into strips, or
  1 lb cod fillet cut into thin slices
4 tsp shoyu
4 tsp brown rice vinegar

Heat the oil in a frying pan. Sprinkle the flour onto a plate. Place the tofu or cod on the flour, coating the top and bottom of each strip. Fry until golden, about 3 minutes, turn over and fry the other side. Put on a serving dish and sprinkle with shoyu and vinegar. Eat immediately.

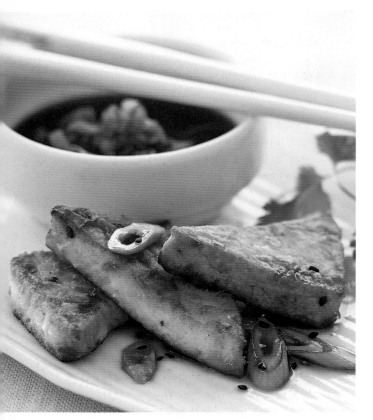

marinated tofu steaks

Light but filling.

 Cooks in 10 minutes, plus marinading

1 block tofu, cut into thin slices
sesame oil
3 tbsp unbleached white flour

FOR THE MARINADE:
1 clove garlic, crushed
1 tsp shichimi
2 small scallions, trimmed and sliced on
  the diagonal
4 tbsp mirin or sake
4 tbsp shoyu
1 tsp black sesame seeds

FOR THE DIPPING SAUCE:
1 tbsp shoyu
1 tsp piece ginger, peeled and finely grated
1 tbsp daikon, grated

Place all the marinade ingredients into a large shallow dish and mix well. Press the tofu in a dry cloth to soak up any liquid. Arrange the tofu slices in the dish, cover and leave at room temperature for 30 minutes. Turn the slices over and marinade for another 30 minutes.

   In another bowl, mix all the dipping sauce ingredients together. Cover and set aside.

   Add just enough oil to coat the bottom of a medium frying pan and heat. Remove the tofu steaks from the marinade and dip in the flour. Cook the steaks, in batches, for 3 minutes each side (you may need to add more oil when cooking subsequent batches.) Drain on kitchen roll and serve with the dipping sauce and any remaining marinade. Eat immediately.

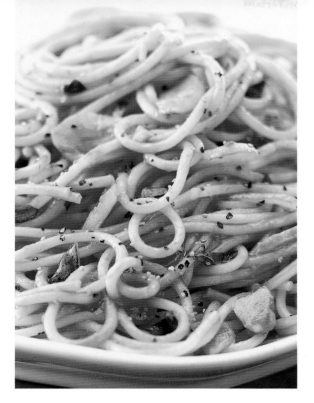

Mediterranean pasta

A quick, energy-boosting dish.

 Cooks in 10 minutes

1 packet organic spagetti
3 tbsp olive oil
1 clove garlic, chopped
sea salt
4 tomatoes, diced
2 tbsp chopped fresh basil, for decoration
12 olives

Cook the pasta according to the packet instructions. Drain and, while still hot, tip into a bowl and add the olive oil and garlic. Mix well. Season with sea salt according to taste and add the tomatoes, olives, and the basil. Eat immediately.

polenta mash

A soothing, creamy dish with strong flavors.

 Cooks in 10 minutes

4 cups rice milk
1 tbsp olive oil
1 tsp sea salt
1 cup polenta (corn grits)
10 black Kalamata olives
½ cup sundried tomatoes, drained and chopped
½ cup mochi, grated
basil leaves, for decoration

Combine the milk, olive oil, and sea salt in a large, heavy-based pan. Bring to a boil. Reduce the heat to low and slowly pour in the polenta, whisking constantly.

After about 3 minutes, add the olives, tomatoes, and mochi. Stir for another minute, then turn off the heat. The mash should be creamy – if it is not, mix in a little more milk. Serve topped with basil leaves. Keeps for 1 day.

shiitake pasta

Rich, satisfying, and filling.

  Cooks in 10 minutes

1 packet organic fusilli pasta
1 tbsp olive oil
1½ cups fresh shiitake mushrooms, sliced
1 bunch scallions, cut into thin, diagonal slices
½ lb organic smoked salmon cut into strips (optional)
½ cup cream
1 tsp sea salt
½ tsp black pepper
2 tbsp fresh flat-leafed parsley, finely chopped, for decoration

Cook the pasta according to the instructions on the packet. When *al dente*, drain and put aside.

Meanwhile, in a large frying pan, heat the oil and add the mushrooms and scallions. Stir-fry for a minute or two. Add 1 tbsp cream, the pasta, fish, salt and black pepper. Toss together well.

Add the rest of the cream and mix thoroughly. Decorate with parsley and serve. Eat immediately.

desserts

nutty rice pudding

A solid dessert that is sweet and relaxing while also providing slow-burning warmth.

  Cooks in 25 minutes

2 cups pre-cooked rice (70% short-grain brown rice, 30% sweet brown rice)
4 cups rice milk (vanilla flavor)
1 cup raisins, washed in warm water
1 medium orange (zest and juice)
3 tbsp maple syrup
ground cinnamon, for decoration
hazelnuts, for garnish

Mix the rice and rice milk together in a medium pan. Bring to a boil, then reduce the heat to medium-low and simmer for 10–15 minutes.

Meanwhile, dry-roast the filberts in a heavy, non-stick frying pan over a low heat, stirring until lightly toasted on all sides (about 2–4 minutes). Roughly chop and use for garnish.

Add the raisins, orange zest, and juice to the rice mixture and simmer for another minute. Add the maple syrup, stir and turn off the heat. Serve the pudding warm in individual bowls, topped with a sprinkle of cinnamon and roasted hazelnuts. Keeps for 1 day.

kanten with pear juice and lemon

A clean-tasting, light, and refreshing dessert.

 Cooks in 5 minutes, plus setting

4 cups natural pear juice
6 heaping tbsp agar-agar
juice of ½ lemon
4 cups of berries, rinsed (optional)

Place the juice and agar agar, together with 2 cups water into a pan and heat gently, stirring continuously. Simmer for three minutes. Turn off the heat and squeeze in the lemon juice.

If you are using berries, place them in a serving bowl and pour the liquid over. Place in the refrigerator and leave to set, gently stirring occasionally to separate the fruit. Otherwise pour into an empty serving bowl. Keeps for 2 days.

hunza apricots with vanilla

The ultimate, naturally sweet dessert.

 Cooks in 30 minutes

32 hunza apricots
1 tbsp arrowroot
juice and rind of ½ lemon
1 cup vanilla rice ice cream (optional) or cream

Soak the apricots in 2 cups cold water overnight. Place the apricots in a 2-quart pan with the soaking water, cover, and bring to a boil. Reduce the heat to medium-low and simmer for about 15–20 minutes. Turn off the heat and leave to stand for 5 minutes.

Remove the apricots with a slotted spoon, then place 8 into each serving bowl. In a cup, dilute the arrowroot with 1 tbsp cold water and add this to the reserved liquid in the pan. Turn the heat back to high and stir constantly for 2 minutes or until the liquid thickens. Turn off the heat and add the lemon juice and rind.

Spoon the liquid over the apricots – there should be about 2 tbsp for each bowl. Finish with a few scoops of vanilla rice ice cream or cream on top. Eat immediately.

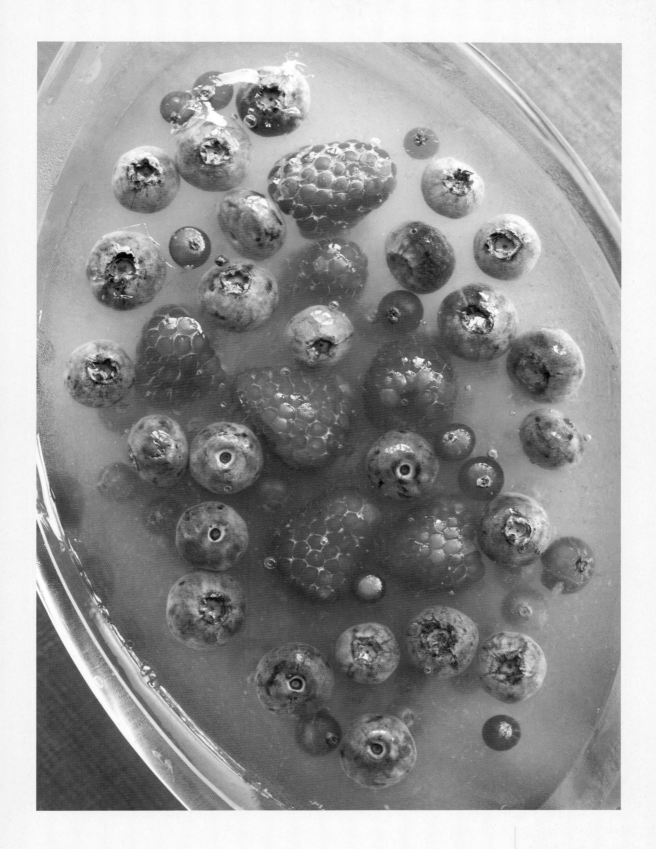

amasake mousse

Helpful when you want to lose yourself in your own thoughts.

  Cooks in 5 minutes

1 cup amasake
1 tbsp kuzu powder
4 tbsp roasted ground almonds
2 tbsp freshly squeezed orange juice
flaked almonds, for decoration
grated ginger (optional)

Put the amasake and ½ cup cold water in a small pan. Measure a further ½ cup cold water in a jug and stir in the kuzu powder. Pour the kuzu mixture into the amasake and slowly bring to a boil, stirring constantly. As the mixture starts to thicken, add the ground almonds. Turn off the heat and stir in the orange juice.

This mousse is delicious warm or at room temperature. Serve garnished with a few flaked almonds. Eat immediately.

stuffed apples

Helps to gently spread your energy.

 Cooks in 25 minutes

½ cup raisins
6 medium-sized apples
3 tbsp tahini
1 tbsp barley miso
1 tsp cinnamon
2 tbsp oil-roasted walnuts, finely chopped
½ cup apple juice (optional)

FOR THE GLAZE:
1 tbsp kuzu
1 tbsp rice syrup

Soak the raisins for 10–15 minutes in a small bowl of hot water. Wash the apples and de-core them.

Use a teaspoon to hollow out the centers of the apples further.

Put the tahini and miso into a bowl and combine with a spoon. Next, stir in the raisins, cinnamon, walnuts, and 1 tbsp water. Fill the apples with the mixture and then place the stuffed apples in a large, deep pan.

Add 1 cup water or a mixture of ½ cup water and ½ cup apple juice, and cover the pan. Bring to a boil, then reduce the heat to medium-low and steam the apples for 10–15 minutes or until they are soft but not mushy. Turn off the heat and remove the apples, reserving the cooking liquid. Place each apple in a serving bowl.

Make the glaze by diluting the kuzu with 1 tbsp cold water and adding it to the liquid in which the apples have been cooked. Gently heat the pan for 2–3 minutes until the kuzu has thickened, stirring constantly to prevent lumps forming. Add the rice syrup to the kuzu mixture, and pour an equal amount of glaze onto each of the apples. Keeps for 1 day.

peach and apple tango

A refreshing dessert that stimulates your upper body.

  Cooks in 15 minutes, plus chilling

4 cups peach and apple juice
pinch of sea salt
4 tbsp kanten or agar-agar flakes
4 sugar-free waffle biscuits (or any other good-quality, sugar-free biscuit)
1 tbsp ready made almond butter
chopped almonds, for decoration

Prepare at least 4 hours before serving. Place the juice in a pan with a pinch of sea salt. Add the kanten or agar-agar flakes and bring to a boil. Simmer for 10 minutes over a medium heat.

Put the waffle biscuits in a deep, flat dish and pour the hot juice over (you can also add any raw chopped fruits, i.e. apples, pears, bananas, or berries, when in season). Leave to cool for a while and then refrigerate for 2–3 hours or until set.

Put 1 tbsp almond butter in a blender and add the juice and biscuit mixture. Blend them all together. Serve the dessert in small dishes, garnished with some chopped almonds. Keeps for 1 day.

stewed fruit

Relaxes your energy, calming your mind.

 Cooks in 20 minutes

4 apples
2 pears or 1 cup raspberries
2 tbsp raisins
organic sugar-free biscuits or waffles (optional)

Put the ingredients (except the biscuits or waffles) and 1 cup water into a pan and simmer together for 15 minutes. Break up the waffles and put into the bottom of the serving bowls. Pour the stewed fruit over and serve. Eat immediately

glazed kuzu pears

A sweet dish that helps you feel content inside.

 Cooks in 20 minutes

2 large or 4 small pears, halved
1 cup pear or apple juice (or a mixture)
pinch of sea salt
4 tsp maple syrup

FOR THE MARZIPAN:
1½ tbsp ground almonds
1 tbsp rice syrup

FOR THE SAUCE:
1 tbsp kuzu powder
1 tbsp lemon juice
1 tsp lemon zest

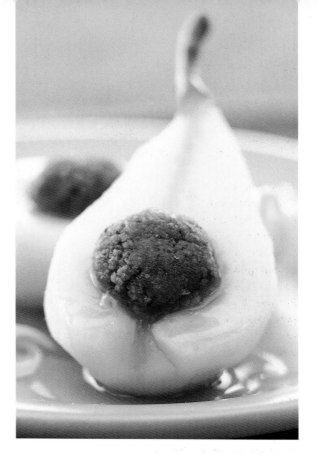

Place the pears (cut side up) and the pear juice in a pan. Bring to a boil. Reduce the heat to medium. Add a pinch of sea salt and cook for 5–7 minutes. Remove the pears using a slotted spoon and reserve the cooking liquid. Place half a pear (or two small halves) in each serving bowl with 1 tsp maple syrup.

Meanwhile, prepare the marzipan. Heat up a frying pan and dry-fry the almonds for 3–5 minutes, stirring constantly. When they are golden brown, remove from the heat.

Heat the rice syrup and add the roasted ground almonds. Mix and stir until the mixture thickens. Place one-quarter of the marzipan in the hollow of each pear half.

In a small pan, mix together the reserved (hot) pear juice and the diluted kuzu powder. Heat, stirring constantly, for 2–3 minutes until the kuzu thickens. Stir in the lemon juice and zest and pour the sauce over the pears to serve. Keeps for 1 day.

summer fruits in syrup

Lifts your spirits and stimulates your mind.

 Cooks in 5 minutes, plus standing

2 cups strawberries
1 cup raspberries
1 cup blueberries
1½ cups strawberry juice, freshly pressed
1 tbsp rum
1 tbsp orange rind
1 tbsp maple syrup
1 tsp ginger, grated
fresh mint leaves, for decoration
soy ice cream (optional)

Wash all the fruits and put them in a large bowl, taking care not to squash them. In another bowl, mix the juice, rum, orange rind, maple syrup, and ginger, and pour this mixture over the fruits. Leave to stand for a couple of hours to allow the flavorings to infuse the fruits.

Serve garnished with mint leaves and soy ice cream, if desired. I like to add a little more orange rind just before serving. Eat immediately.

coffee mousse

A dessert with bite that helps free your mind.

 Cooks in 20 minutes, plus chilling

4 cups organic sugar-free apple juice
5 tbsp instant Yannoh coffee
6 tbsp agar-agar
1 tsp natural vanilla extract
2 tbsp smooth organic peanut butter
3 tbsp rice syrup
dry-roasted walnuts, finely chopped, for decoration

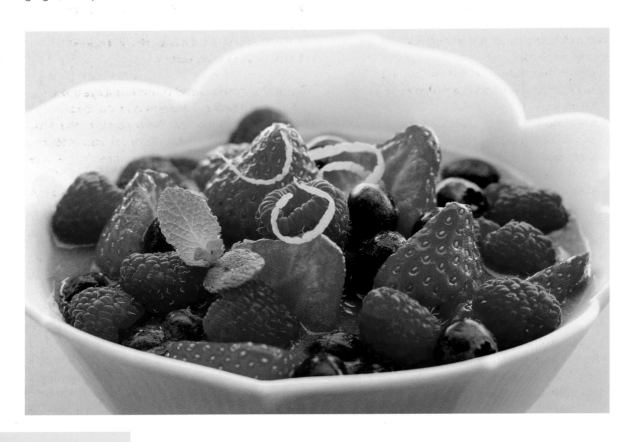

Place the apple juice with 2 cups cold water in a large pan and bring to a boil. Put the Yannoh in a cup, add a few tbsp water and mix into a smooth paste. Add the paste and agar-agar flakes to the apple juice and water mixture, and stir well. Cook for 10 minutes on a medium heat until the agar-agar completely dissolves.

Turn off the heat and pour into a large dish. Leave to cool for 15 minutes and then refrigerate for about an hour or until the mixture has set.

Once set, put the mousse into a blender with the vanilla extract, peanut butter, and syrup, and process until smooth. Spoon into 4 bowls and chill for 5 minutes. Decorate with a sprinkling of chopped walnuts. Keeps for 1 day.

nutty strudel

A satisfying dessert that settles your energy.

  Cooks in 50 minutes

6–8 eating apples, peeled and grated
3 tbsp maple syrup
½ cup walnuts, lightly roasted and ground
½ cup raisins, washed and soaked in hot water for
   10 minutes
1 tbsp whole-grain bread crumbs
1 packet fresh phyllo pastry
2 tbsp olive oil
3–4 tbsp sparkling mineral water
1 cup natural vanilla custard

Preheat the oven to 350°F. In a mixing bowl, mix the apples, maple syrup, walnuts, raisins, and bread crumbs together.

Unroll 4 sheets of phyllo pastry. Put 1 sheet on the worktop, sprinkle with a few drops of corn oil and brush it all over the pastry. Cover with another piece of phyllo and a little more oil. Repeat with all 4 sheets. Put 3 or 4 tablespoons of the apple filling in the center of the pastry and roll it up like a Swiss roll. Repeat until you have used up all the phyllo and the filling.

Place the rolls on a baking tray. Drizzle with some more oil and bake for about 20–25 minutes. Turn the oven off. Take the rolls out of the oven and sprinkle with mineral water (this stops the pastry from drying out).

Put the rolls back in the oven, without turning it on again, and leave for 5 minutes. Make the vanilla custard according to the packet instructions. Cut the strudels into pieces and serve with the custard poured over. Keeps for 1 day.

chestnut balls

A rich, filling dessert that slowly energizes your lower abdomen.

 Cooks in 1 hour 15 minutes, plus soaking

2 cups dried chestnuts
½ cup adzuki beans
2 cups sugar-free fruit juice (any kind you like)
½ cup raisins
½ cup dry roasted hazelnuts, finely chopped
1 cup natural vanilla custard

Place the chestnuts and beans in a large bowl, cover with the fruit juice and leave to soak overnight. Next day, put the contents of the bowl in a pressure-cooker with the raisins and cook for 45 minutes. Turn the heat off, reduce the pressure slowly, uncover and leave to cool.

Use a slotted spoon to take the chestnuts out of the cooker. Remove any remaining skin, as this tends to be bitter. Put all the ingredients in a blender and process, or simply mash them with a fork. With moistened hands, form the mixture into balls the size of golf balls – you should end up with about 12 balls. Roll these in the chopped hazelnuts. Make the vanilla custard according to the packet instructions and serve. Keeps for 1 day.

broken cookie crumble

Helps to bring your energy down and makes you feel more relaxed and settled.

 Cooks in 35 minutes

4 organic apples, peeled and coarsely chopped
4 organic pears, peeled and coarsely chopped
juice of 2 medium-sized organic oranges
1 tbsp sugar-free peach jam
½ cup rice syrup
½ packet plain, sugar-free cookies
½ cup flaked almonds

Preheat the oven to 350°F. Place the chopped apples and pears in an ovenproof dish. In a small mixing bowl, stir together the orange juice, jam, and syrup and pour the mixture over the fruit.

Wrap the cookies in a large cotton tea towel and then crush them to fine crumbs with a rolling pin. Sprinkle the cookie crumbs over the fruit and scatter the flaked almonds on top. Bake for 20–25 minutes. Keeps for 2 days.

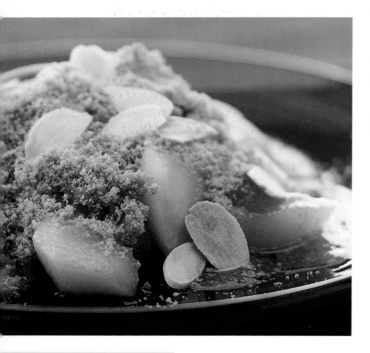

almond and hazelnut cookies

A satisfying snack.

  Cooks in 40 minutes

½ cup almonds
½ cup hazelnuts
1 cup whole-wheat pastry flour
1 cup white unbleached flour
1 tbsp salt-free baking powder
½ cup apple juice
½ cup maple syrup
½ tsp vanilla extract
oil, for greasing
sugar-free jam (optional)

Preheat the oven to 350°F. To dry-roast the almonds and hazelnuts, place them in a heavy-based, non-stick frying pan and stir over a low heat for 2–4 minutes until lightly toasted on all sides. Cool and roughly chop the roasted nuts.

Mix the flours and baking powder together in a bowl. Add the almonds and hazelnuts. In a blender, mix together the apple juice, maple syrup, and vanilla extract. Pour over the flour mixture. Stir to form a smooth dough, adding more flour if necessary.

On a lightly floured worktop, roll out the dough to about ½-inch thickness. Using cookie cutters, cut out different shapes and place onto a lightly oiled baking tray. Bake for 15–20 minutes. If you've got a very sweet tooth, serve topped with some sugar-free jam. Keeps for 2 days.

pancakes

Fills your abdomen with long-lasting fuel.

  Cooks in 20 minutes, plus chilling

MAKES ABOUT 20 PANCAKES:
2 cups organic whole-wheat pastry flour
pinch of sea salt
1 tsp kuzu powder
2 cups beer or cold sparkling mineral water
1 tbsp olive oil, plus extra for cooking

Preheat the oven to 200°F. Mix the flour and sea salt together in a mixing bowl. Dilute the kuzu in a few tbsp beer or water and stir until it dissolves. Make a well in the middle and gradually add the kuzu and some more of the beer or water, stirring constantly. When you have added 1 cup of the liquid, the mixture should form a wet but firm dough. Pound with a wooden spoon for 5 minutes, making sure there are no lumps. Thin the dough down with the remaining water or beer until it is more like a batter, and stir well. Leave it in the refrigerator for 15 minutes.

Stir 1 tbsp of the oil into the batter. Pour ¼ tsp of the oil into a medium-sized, heavy-based frying pan and heat over a high heat. Pour in one ladleful of batter, swirling the pan as you pour, to ensure the base of the pan is covered with batter. Cook for 1–2 minutes until the batter is set and just starting to turn golden on the base. Flip the pancake over using a palette knife and cook the other side for 2 minutes. Repeat with the remaining batter to make about 20 pancakes. Keep them warm in the oven while you cook the remainder.

Serve the pancakes warm with your favorite sugar-free jam, or maple syrup and lemon juice. Eat immediately.

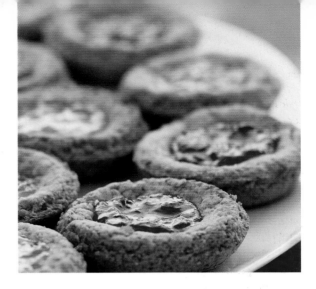

jam tarts

A good snack for feeling grounded.

  Cooks in 35 minutes

MAKES 15–20 TARTS:
3 cups organic whole-wheat pastry flour
¼ tsp sea salt
½ cup corn oil
½ cup maple syrup
4–6 tbsp sparkling mineral water (or enough to make a dough)
sugar-free jam of your choice

Preheat the oven to 350°F. Combine the flour and sea salt in a mixing bowl. Mix the oil and the syrup in a jug and then add it to the flour. Slowly add enough water to form a dough. Knead lightly for a minute. Try not to work the dough too much or it will be tough; it should remain powdery. Put the dough in the freezer for 5 minutes.

Remove the dough from the freezer. Spread a little flour over the worktop and gently roll out the dough to a ½-inch thickness.

Using a small round pastry cutter, stamp out 15 or so rounds. Place each pastry circle in a muffin tray, and make a little depression in the pastry with your thumb. Fill each with ½ tsp of jam. Bake in the oven for 15–20 minutes. Keeps for 3 days.

teas and infusions

green and brown rice tea

Can be helpful in reducing cholesterol

  Cooks in 5 minutes

**4 tsp green and brown rice
tea mixture**

Boil 4 cups water and let it stand for 2 minutes.
Put the tea leaves and roasted rice in a teapot and
pour the water over them. Let it stand for a few
minutes more before serving. The water needs to
be hot to produce the desired taste and the lovely
light color of the green tea.

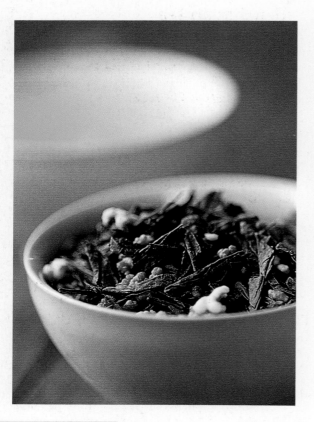

bancha twig tea

*Contains less caffeine than ordinary tea and is good
for digestive problems.*

 Cooks in 5 minutes

1 tbsp bancha twigs

Place the twigs and 4 cups water in a pan. Bring to
the boil then turn off. Leave for several minutes
and serve.

sweet vegetable tea

A relaxing, re-energizing tea.

 Cooks in 20 minutes

¼ cup onions, cut into half-moons
¼ cup carrots, cut into matchsticks
¼ cup cabbage, shredded
¼ cup parsnips, cut into matchsticks

Bring 3 cups water to a boil, then lower the heat
and add all the vegetables. Simmer for 15–20
minutes, covered. Strain and drink one cup while
hot. Let the remaining tea cool down before
storing it in the refrigerator. Each time you have a
cup of this tea, warm up one serving in a pot to
room temperature.

parsley tea

A stimulating and mind-energizing tea.

  Cooks in 5 minutes

¼ cup parsley, finely chopped

Place the parsley and 1 cup water in a small pan.
Bring to a boil, reduce the flame and simmer for
10 minutes. Strain and drink while hot.

umeboshi bancha tea

Good for digestive troubles and fatigue.

 Cooks in 5 minutes

bancha twig tea (see left)
¼–½ umeboshi (depending on size)
½ tsp shoyu

Put the umeboshi and then the shoyu in a cup.
Pour over the hot bancha twig tea and drink
while warm.

dried daikon tea

*This tea is perfect if you need to relax. It is
also thought to be helpful in ridding the body
of saturated fats.*

  Cooks in 15 minutes

½ cup dried daikon

Place 3 cups water in a pan and add the dried
daikon. Cover the pan and bring to the boil.
Reduce the heat to medium-low and simmer for 20
minutes. Strain and serve.

It is a good idea to make enough tea for 3–4
servings and have 1 cup a day. Refrigerate any
leftover tea and reheat it before drinking.

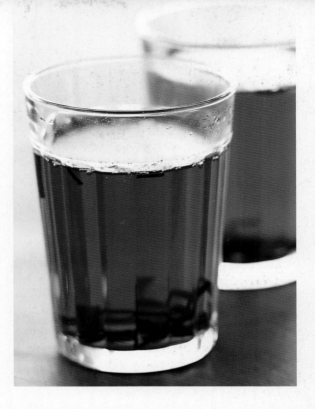

adzuki bean tea

*The energy of this tea strengthens kidney energy and
can help with kidney-related problems.*

  Cooks in 35 minutes

½ cup adzuki beans
1-inch piece kombu

Put the beans, kombu, and 3 cups water into a
pan, cover, and bring to a boil. Reduce the heat to
very low and simmer, covered, for about 30
minutes. Strain and drink.

You may like to make enough tea for a few days,
keep it refrigerated and use one cup at a time
slightly warmed up. Keep the beans and use them
in dishes such as soups, stews, and casseroles.
Make sure you cook them further until they are
soft and edible.

shiitake tea

Said to be good for eliminating fats from the body.

 Cooks in 25 minutes

**2 medium-sized dried shiitake
mushrooms**
¼ tsp shoyu

Soak the mushrooms in ½ cup cold water until soft (this should take 10–15 minutes). Cut off and discard the stems and slice the caps. Put the mushrooms and 2 cups water (including the soaking water) into a pan.

Cover and bring to the boil. Reduce the heat to medium-low and simmer for 5 minutes. Add the shoyu and turn off the heat. Leave to stand for a couple of minutes, then strain and serve.

shoyu bancha with scallion drink

If you are getting a cold or flu, drink this tea as hot as possible. It is also believed to increase your resistance to infection.

  Cooks in 5 minutes

1 tsp shoyu
1 small scallion, very finely chopped diagonally
bancha twig tea (see page 154)

Place the shoyu and scallion in a cup. Pour the hot bancha twig tea over. Drink as hot as possible.

agar-agar drink

Although, unlike other sea vegetables, agar-agar does not contain many nutrients, it is very helpful in cases of acute or even chronic constipation.

  Cooks in 15 minutes

1 cup sugar-free organic apple juice
sea salt
1 tbsp agar-agar

Combine the apple juice, a pinch of sea salt, and the agar-agar in a small pan. Cover and bring to the boil. Reduce the heat to medium-low and simmer for 10 minutes. Drink hot.

lemon and ginger tea

An expansive, stimulating tea.

 Cooks in 5 minutes

½ lemon
1 tsp fresh ginger, grated

Squeeze the lemon juice into a glass and add the grated ginger. Add boiling water and slices of lemon to intensify the flavor. Drink while hot.

mint tea

An "up," refreshing drink.

 Cooks in 5 minutes

6 medium-sized fresh mint leaves

Put the mint leaves in a cup and pour over boiling water. Leave to steep for 3 minutes before drinking.

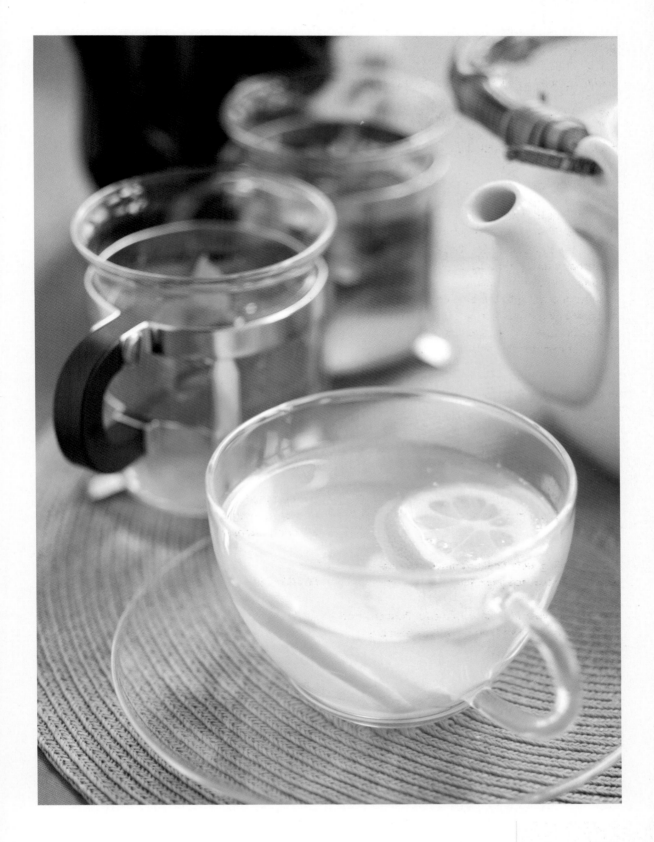

index

acknowledgments

I feel enormous appreciation to Michio and Aveline Kushi for their incredible generosity of spirit in giving me so much so freely and for their immeasurable contribution to the macrobiotic movement. I have always cherished my time spent with them. Michio I admire you and I hope history will judge you to be a very special person.

Thank you to Melanie and Denny Waxman for being instrumental in getting me started. Dragana I love all those delicious macro meals you whipped up when it was the last thing on your agenda. Christopher, Alexander, Nicholas, and Michael for being so tolerant "Oh, dad! Not brown rice, bean, natto, nishime pumpkin, and steamed greens again!"

I have always found the macrobiotic crowd at large to be stimulating and without naming names (due to shortage of space) I would like to thank all those I have met over the years for their wonderful contribution.

Picture credits:
Getty Images/Food Pix jacket and page 118
Getty Images page 112
Photolibrary pages 93 and 116

Simon began his career in macrobiotics in 1980, initially attending classes at The East West Center in London. In 1984 he went to America where he studied with Michio and Aveline Kushi, Shizuko Yamamoto, Denny Waxman, Bill Tara, and many other macrobiotic teachers. Simon went on to run the Macrobiotic Association of Philadelphia.

In 1986 Simon was invited to return to London to run the East West Center. At the time this was Europe's largest alternative health center, where you could learn anything from Tai Chi to Acupuncture. Here Simon organized professional macrobiotic courses and Michio and Aveline as well as Shizuko regularly led courses.

Since 1993 Simon has written numerous books including those on feng shui, face reading, chi energy, do in exercise, and astrology. Simon is also involved in the London health food store Luscious Organic.

CONSULTATIONS WITH SIMON
Simon provides individual macrobiotic health consultations, either in person or by phone or email, in which he will help design a specific macrobiotic diet to suit each person and provide support in getting started.

CONTACT SIMON
Phone: +44 (0) 20 7431 9897
Email: simon@chienergy.co.uk
Website: www.chienergy.co.uk

USEFUL WEBSITES
www.celebrate4health.com
www.chienergy.co.uk
www.cybermacro.com
www.e-macrobiotica.com
www.healingcuisine.com
www.kushiinstitute.org
www.lusciousorganic.co.uk
www.macroamerica.com
www.macrobiotics.co.uk
www.macrobiotics.org.uk
www.michaelrossoff.com
www.natural-connection.com
www.organic-food-london.com
www.phiya.com
www.strengthenhealth.org
www.whfoods.com
www.worldmacro.org